THE 50 RECIPES ON ITALIAN VEGETARIAN CUISINE PASTA, PIZZA AND SOUPS 2021/22

If you love the Italian cuisine you can't miss the famous first courses that come from the culinary recipes of every Italian region, Pasta, Pizza and Soups a complete recipe book both to lose weight but also satisfy your sins of gluttony.

Alfredo Savona

ALFREDO SAVONA

THE 50 RECIPES ON ITALIAN VEGETARIAN CUISINE PASTA, PIZZA AND SOUPS 2021/22

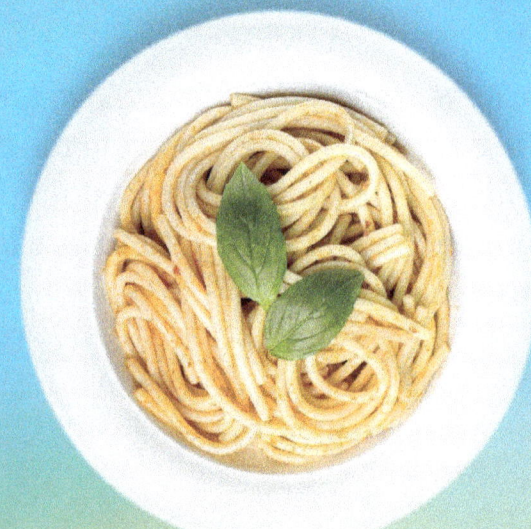

IF YOU LOVE THE ITALIAN CUISINE YOU CAN'T MISS THE FAMOUS FIRST COURSES THAT COME FROM THE CULINARY RECIPES OF EVERY ITALIAN REGION, PASTA, PIZZA AND SOUPS A COMPLETE RECIPE BOOK BOTH TO LOSE WEIGHT BUT ALSO SATISFY YOUR SINS OF GLUTTONY.

Table of Contents

INTRODUCTION 10

1. CREAMY ASPARAGUS RISOTTO 12
2. VEGETARIAN TOFU BOLOGNESE 14
3. PERFECT PIZZA PANCAKES 16
4. ITALIAN TUSCAN VEGETABLE SOUP 18
5. ROASTED EGGPLANT PARMESAN STACKS 20
6. EASY TOMATO SPINACH PASTA 23
7. SIMPLE SOCCA PIZZA RECIPE 25
8. CREAMY PESTO GNOCCHI 27
9. VEGAN MUSHROOM RISOTTO 29
10. CHEESE BAKED RIGATONI WITH ROASTED VEGETABLES 31
11. PASTA ARRABIATA 34
12. COMFORTING LEEK RISOTTO 36
13. RED PESTO PASTA 39
14. VEGETARIAN ZUCCHINI 41
15. CRISPY TORTILLA PIZZA 43
16. LEMON PAPPARDELLE 45
17. SMOKY BAKED EGGS WITH RICOTTA AND BEANS 47

18. CREAMY BROCCOLI PASTA 49

19. ITALIAN SUMMER VEGETABLE CASSEROLE 51

20. CREAMY AVOCADO PASTA 54

21. BROWN RICE RISOTTO WITH BUTTERNUT SQUASH & MUSHROOMS 56

22. SPAGHETTI CACIO E PEPE 59

23. ITALIAN TORTELLINI SPINACH SOUP 62

24. TOMATO MOZZARELLA BREAD 64

25. CAPRESE SALAD 66

26. ITALIAN SAUTEED SWISS CHARD 68

27. THE BRUSCHETTA 70

28. VERZA STUFATA 72

29. ITALIAN VEGETARIAN STUFFED MUSHROOMS 74

30. HOMEMADE BASIL PESTO 78

31. EGGPLANT ROLLATINI 80

32. HOMEMADE RAVIOLI 83

33. LINGUINE WITH FRESH TOMATOES 86

34. CHERRY TOMATO & BASIL FOCACCIA 88

35. TORTELLINI WITH TOMATO SPINACH CREAM SAUCE 91

36. EGGPLANT PARMESAN 93

37. GRILLED BRUSCHETTA 95

38. MAKE-AHEAD SPINACH MANICOTTI 97

39. ARTICHOKE CAPRESE PLATTER 99

40. GNOCCHI ALFREDO 101

41. CREAMY ITALIAN POTATO SALAD 103

42. PANZANELLA PASTA 106

43. BOW TIES WITH WALNUT-HERB PESTO 108

44. MUSHROOM BOLOGNESE WITH WHOLE WHEAT PASTA 110

45. ITALIAN-STYLE PIZZAS 112

46. CREAMY PASTA PRIMAVERA 114

47. TUSCAN PORTOBELLO STEW 116

48. SLOW-COOKER CAPONATA 118

49. GNOCCHI WITH MUSHROOMS AND ONION 120

50. QUINOA ARANCINI 122

CONCLUSION 124

© Copyright 2021 by Alfredo Savona - All rights reserved.

The following Book is reproduced below with the goal of providing information that is as accurate and reliable as possible. Regardless, purchasing this Book can be seen as consent to the fact that both the publisher and the author of this book are in no way experts on the topics discussed within and that any recommendations or suggestions that are made herein are for entertainment purposes only. Professionals should be consulted as needed prior to undertaking any of the action endorsed herein.

This declaration is deemed fair and valid by both the American Bar Association and the Committee of Publishers Association and is legally binding throughout the United States.

Furthermore, the transmission, duplication, or reproduction of any of the following work including specific information will be considered an illegal act irrespective of if it is done electronically or in print. This extends to creating a secondary or tertiary copy of the work or a recorded copy and is only allowed with the express written consent from the Publisher. All additional right reserved.

The information in the following pages is broadly considered a truthful and accurate account of facts and as such, any inattention, use, or misuse of the information in question by the reader will render any resulting actions solely under their purview. There are no scenarios in which the publisher or the original author of this work can be in any fashion deemed liable for any hardship or damages that may befall them after undertaking information described herein.

Additionally, the information in the following pages is intended only for informational purposes and should thus be thought of as universal. As befitting its nature, it is presented without assurance regarding its prolonged validity or interim quality. Trademarks that are mentioned are done without written consent and can in no way be considered an endorsement from the trademark holder.

☆ *55% OFF for BookStore NOW at $ 30,95 instead of $ 41,95!* ☆

Welcome to Italian Vegetarian Cuisine,

considered the most important Cuisine in Europe and maybe even in the world.

That's why if you are a lover of vegetarian cuisine, you cannot miss the recipes described in this book.

Good life and good appetite, my friends.

Buy is NOW and let your Customers get addicted to this amazing book!

INTRODUCTION

Italian vegetarian cuisine is so much more than just risotto (although, with so many regions growing rice across the country, it's certainly a dish Italians know how to make well).

From the truffles of Tuscany to the plump, fragrant tomatoes of Campania, Italy's regions all offer their own unique products that lend themselves perfectly to the creation of a whole host of imaginative vegetarian dishes.

It's no surprise then that the best vegetarian restaurants in Europe are in Italy, so many have already received a Michelin star.

In this cookbook, I propose many vegetarian recipes revisited by me, taking inspiration from the best Italian recipes scattered in many regions.

Build your favorite dishes and improve your culinary skills more and more.

Create a vegetarian dinner party menu that's full of surprises with this collection of ingenious vegetarian Italian recipes, all of which demonstrate the versatility and imagination of Italy's greatest chefs.

Start as you mean to go on with the recipes, a superb vegetarian beginner dish made from auberge, herbs and a striking charcoal mayonnaise, or try his equally colorful Butterfly salad, featuring radicchio, green cabbage, carrots, spinach and beetroot to create a veritable vegetarian feast for all the senses.

Let's start.

1. Creamy Asparagus Risotto

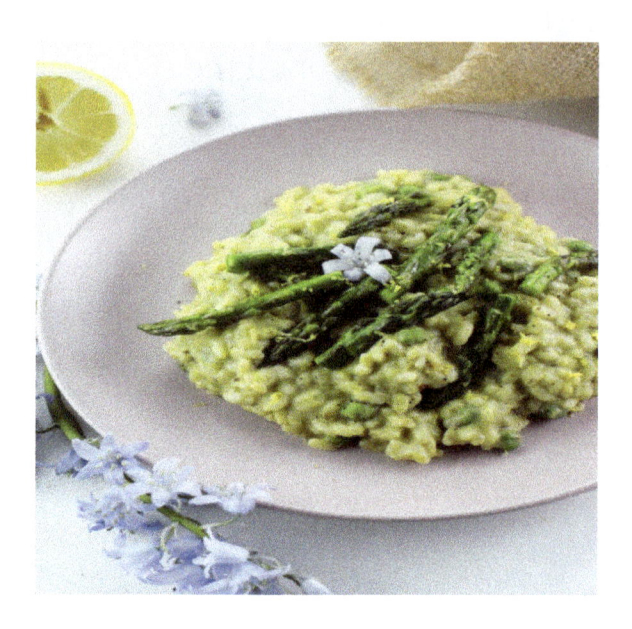

Ingredients

½ cup risotto rice (Carnaroli gives the best results but Arborio is easier to find)
1 handful asparagus
1 tbsp butter (or double the amount olive oil)
1 small onion
1 cup peas (fresh, canned or frozen are fine)
3 cups vegetable broth
½ cup hard cheese, grated

Direction

Cut the asparagus into small pieces.
Finely dice the onion.
Melt the butter and oil in a frying pan, add the onion and fry until translucent.
Add the rice and fry for a minute or two. (Optional: fry the rice in 1/2 cup of white wine until the wine evaporates).
Then add 500 ml of broth and stir.
Leave to simmer for 15 minutes on low heat (preferably nearby so you can stir occasionally).
Add the asparagus and peas, stir and leave for a further 5 minutes.
You may need to add a little more liquid (this will depend on the heat).
Now check the rice. It may need a few more minutes to finish cooking.
When the rice is soft, it's time to finish it - add a little water if necessary (add it in small amounts, you don't want to overdo it!) and a little grated cheese to give it a creamy taste.
Remember: it must flow like lava.

2. Vegetarian Tofu Bolognese

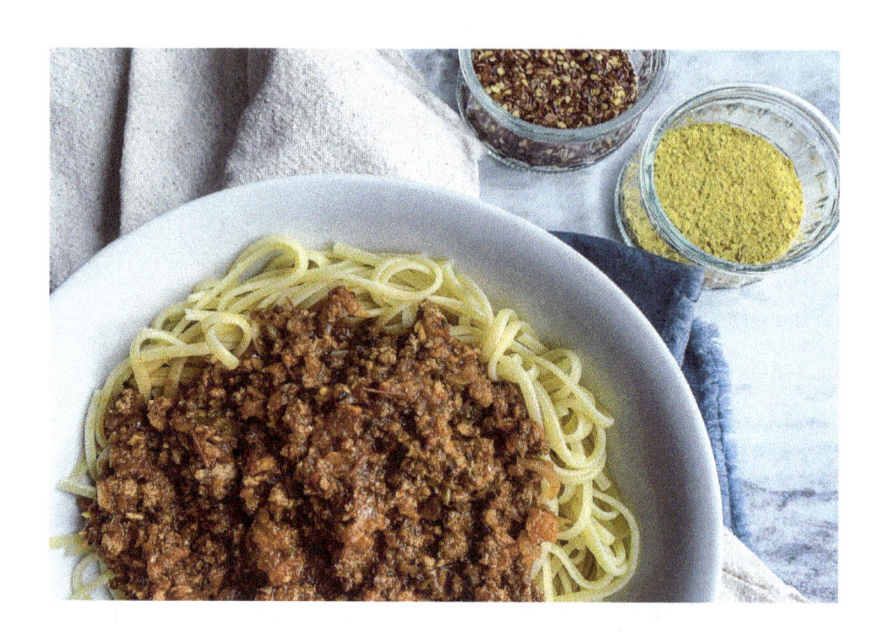

Ingredients

For the pasta
7 oz whole wheat pasta (choose your favourite, wholegrain would be best)
1 tsp olive oil
For the tofu
7 oz firm tofu (ideally get fresh tofu from the supermarket)
1 tsp olive oil
For the sauce
1 tsp olive oil
1 red onion
2 clove garlic

1 can diced tomatoes (1 can = 14.5 oz)
2 tbsp tomato paste
1 handful basil, fresh (or 2 tbsp frozen or dry basil)
1 tsp oregano, dried
1 tsp maple syrup (or brown sugar)
salt and pepper to taste

Direction

For pasta
Cook the pasta as directed. Drizzle the prepared pasta with olive oil to taste, add a little salt and oregano.
For the sauce
Dice the onion and garlic.
Heat the oil in a frying pan and add the onion and garlic. Fry for 3-4 minutes. Now add the chopped tomatoes, tomato paste, basil, maple syrup, salt and pepper. Allow to simmer.
Tofu
Cut the tofu into small pieces or crumble it to resemble mince.
In a large frying pan, heat the oil to medium heat and add the tofu. Add a little salt and leave to fry for 15 minutes or until crispy. Be sure to stir occasionally, have patience and taste! If you crumble it, reduce the cooking time by about 3 min.
When everything is ready, add the pasta to the plate, pour the sauce on top and add the tofu.

3. Perfect Pizza Pancakes

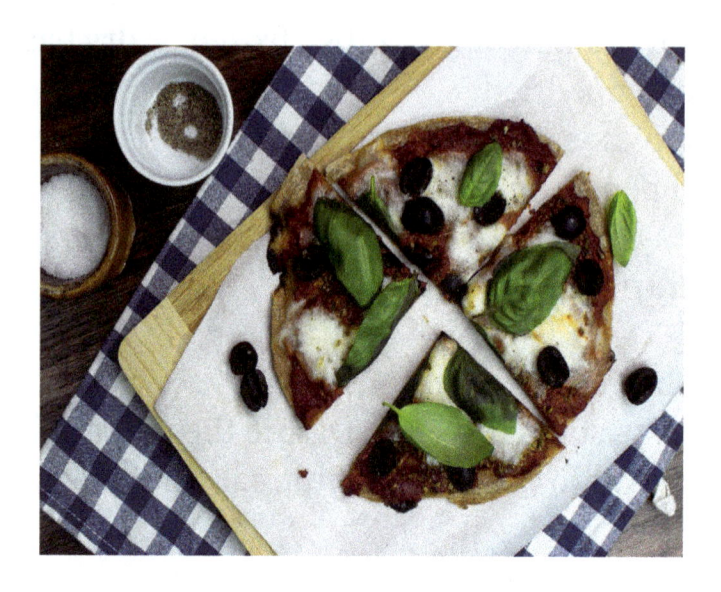

Ingredients

¾ cup flour (¾ cup = 130g)
⅔ cup water (⅔ cup = 150ml)
1 tsp olive oil
1 tsp dried yeast
3 tbsp tomato paste (thick stuff)
2 tbsp dried Italian herbs (or oregano)
1 ball low fat mozzarella (1 ball = 125g/4.5oz)(use regular if you prefer)
8 olives
1 handful basil leaves, fresh

Direction

Mix the yeast, water and flour until smooth.
Pour into a lightly oiled frying pan. Spread the batter evenly. There is enough dough for two small or one large pizza.
Give it a minute or two to set, then turn it over. For best results, bake with the lid on.
Add the tomato paste and the dried herbs. Spread evenly over the base.
Slice the mozzarella and olives and place them on top.
Bake with the lid on. 8-10 minutes for thin and crispy, 15 minutes for deep frying.
Add fresh basil at the end.

4. Italian Tuscan Vegetable Soup

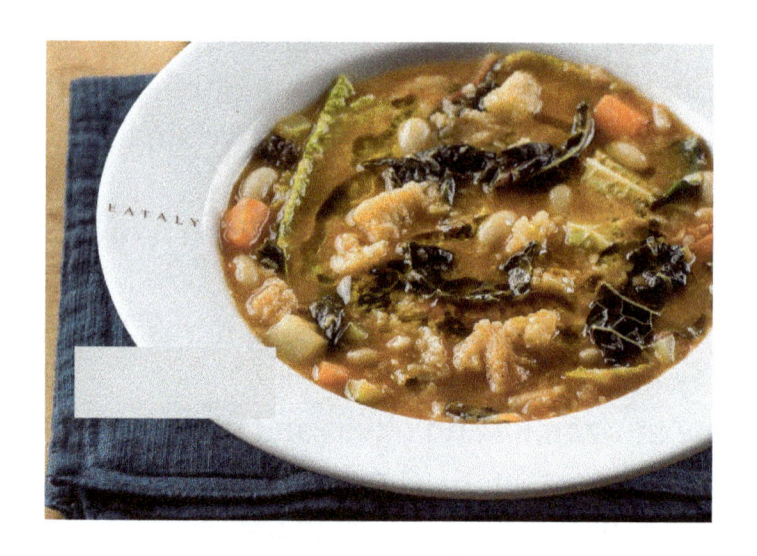

Ingredients

2 Tbsp. Olive Oil
6 cloves Garlic
1 Onion (any color)
2-3 stalks Celery
1 Bell Pepper (any color)
3-4 cups Green Beans (washed and trimmed)
6 cups Gluten Free Vegetable Broth
1 14 oz. can Diced Tomatoes
1 tsp. Italian Seasoning
2 15 oz. cans Kidney Beans (drained and rinsed)
1.5 cups Gluten Free Rotini Noodles (can use regular noodles if not GF)
¼ tsp. Kosher Salt and Pepper

2-3 cups chopped Kale
Parmesan Cheese for garnish

Direction

Mince 6 cloves of garlic and 1 onion (any colour). Cut 2-3 celery stalks into small slices.
Dice 1 bell pepper of any colour.
Wash and trim 1 pound of green beans. Cut the beans in halves or thirds, depending on the size you like them.
Preheat a cast-iron Dutch oven or heavy-bottomed soup pan on the stove to medium or medium-high.
When the oil is hot, add the chopped garlic, onion and celery. Fry for 2-3 minutes, stirring frequently.
Add the chopped green beans, a pinch of salt and pepper and fry for 4-5 minutes, stirring frequently.
Add the diced peppers and fry for a further 2-3 minutes, stirring frequently.
The vegetables should smell nice when fried in oil.
If you want more soups to help you warm up this winter, be sure to check out this winter root vegetable soup, lentil sausage soup, slow-cooked chicken potato soup, butternut sausage soup and slow-cooked turkey chili.

5. Roasted Eggplant Parmesan Stacks

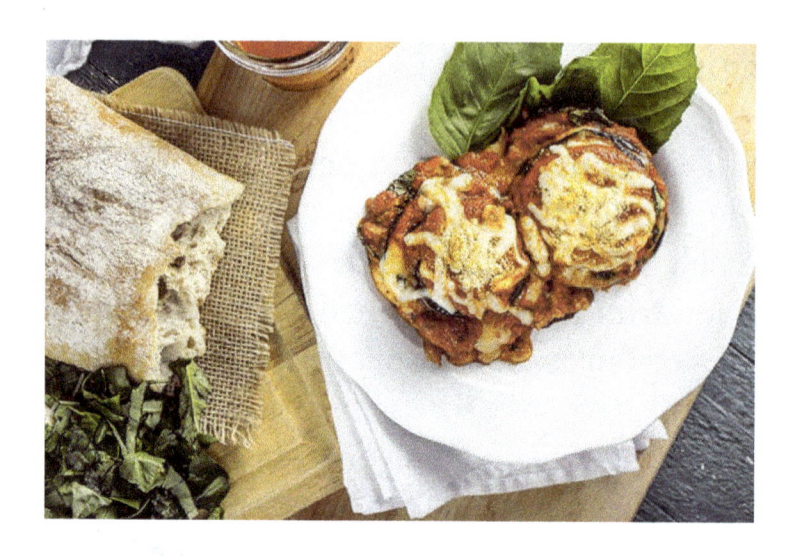

Ingredients

12 slices of aubergine about 1/2 inch thick (about 1 large aubergine)
4 tablespoons extra virgin olive oil
kosher salt to taste
black pepper to taste
1 cup prepared or homemade marinara sauce
8 ounces fresh mozzarella, cut into 12 slices (see notes)
3/4 cup grated Parmesan cheese (see notes)
1/4 cup fresh basil cut into chiffons
more olive oil, Parmesan cheese, fresh cracked pepper and/or crushed red pepper (optional)

Direction

Preheat the oven to 425 degrees Celsius.
Arrange the aubergine slices on a baking sheet and brush them front and back with all 4 tablespoons of olive oil. Coat quickly as the eggplant will absorb the oil. Season generously on both sides with kosher salt and black pepper.
Bake the aubergine slices at 425 degrees for 30-40 minutes until well cooked and browned.
Remove all but four baked eggplant slices to a plate. Arrange the remaining four on the baking sheet to distribute evenly.
Place a spoonful (slightly more than a spoonful) of the marinara sauce on top of the four aubergine slices. Place a slice of fresh mozzarella and about a tablespoon of grated Parmesan cheese, followed by a few pieces of fresh basil.
Repeat the layers two more times, but do not add fresh basil in the last layer. You will now have four piles of three aubergine slices each.
Bake at 425 degrees for 10 minutes or until the cheese melts.
When you take it out of the oven, sprinkle the remaining basil on top of each pile (this is added after baking to prevent it from drying out and burning).
Serve with a drizzle of pure olive oil, more Parmesan cheese, fresh cracked black pepper and, if necessary, a little crushed red pepper.

6. Easy Tomato Spinach Pasta

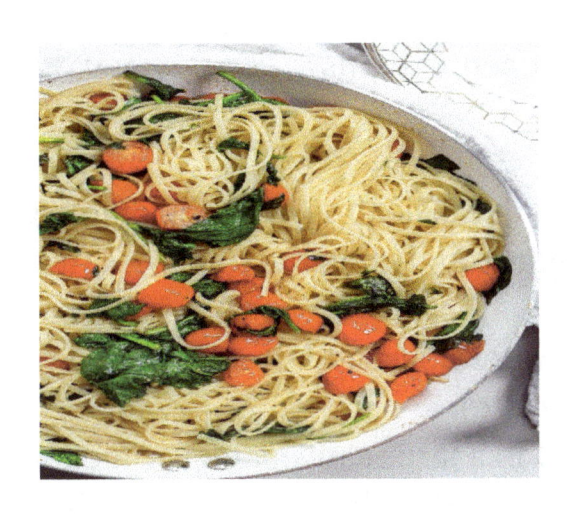

Ingredients

2 cups penne pasta
3 tbsp olive oil
1 small onion
2 cloves of garlic
4 small tomatoes (4 fresh tomatoes = 1 can of diced tomatoes)
2 tablespoons tomato paste
3-4 tbsp Greek yoghurt (or cream cheese if you want to be naughty)
1 large handful of spinach (1 large handful = 200 g, frozen spinach is fine)
¼ cup grated hard cheese
1 teaspoon dried oregano

1 tsp dried basil
1 pinch of red pepper flakes
½ teaspoon salt
½ teaspoon peppercorns

Direction

While the water is heating, dice the onion, grate or crush the garlic and chop the tomatoes (if not using a can).
When the water boils, add the pasta (add salt and a little oil to taste).
Heat the oil in a large saucepan over medium heat, add the onion and garlic and fry for 5 minutes or until translucent.
Add the tomatoes. Note: if you use fresh tomatoes, the sauce will be a little runny. Only if you let it stand for a day will you get the creamy texture you are looking for.
Add the spinach.
Add oregano, basil, red pepper flakes, salt and pepper.
Stir in the tomato paste and Greek yoghurt. Stir until both are dissolved in the sauce.
Now add the hard cheese.
Drain and add the pasta. Reduce the heat to simmer. Stir occasionally for 1 minute. Taste and adjust the salt and pepper if necessary.

7. Simple Socca Pizza Recipe

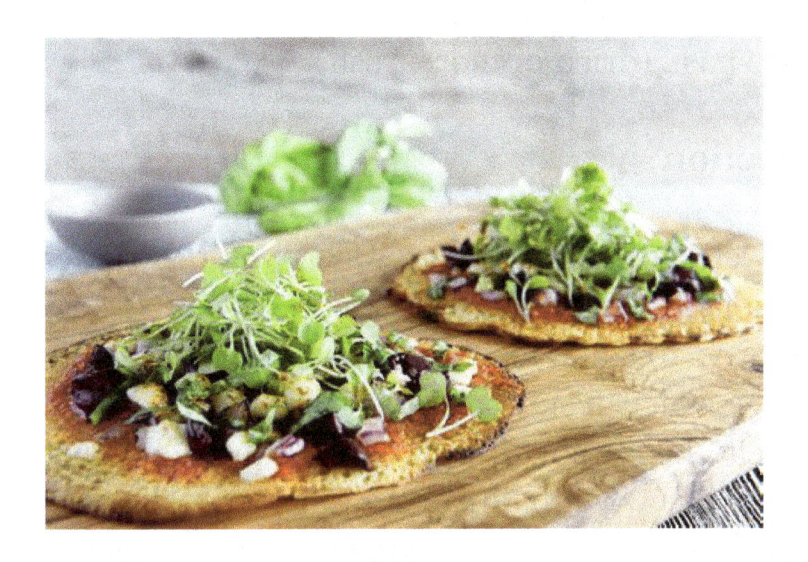

Ingredients

Pizza base:
1 cup chickpea flour: 1 cup chickpea flour
1 cup warm water
½ teaspoon garlic powder
1 teaspoon baking powder
1 tbsp oil
Pinch of salt
Stuffing:
Seasoning. We like:
4 tbsp tomato paste (thick)
1-2 tablespoons dried oregano
1 small red onion
1 cup cheddar cheese (grated)

½ cup sweetcorn
1 handful of olives
1 handful of rocket (arugula)
1 tbsp basil (dried or more fresh)

Direction

Mix well the chickpea flour, warm water, garlic powder and baking powder. For best results, cover and leave to stand for thirty minutes. If you are short of time, you can skip this step.
Preheat the oven to 200 °C/390 °F and mix the olive oil with the wet mixture and a pinch of salt.
Pour the mixture into a baking tray with sides and parchment paper. Allow to bake for about 8 minutes, until it starts to firm up a little.
Thinly slice the red onion and prepare the cheese, olives and corn.
Remove the pizza base from the oven and brush it with tomato paste and sprinkle with dried oregano. Layer the other ingredients on top, including basil or your favourite herbs, with the exception of the arugula/rocket, which we now wash and drain.
Bake for about 12 minutes more. When everything looks ready and the cheese has melted, the pizza is ready! Remove from the oven and decorate with arugula and/or rocket.

8. Creamy Pesto Gnocchi

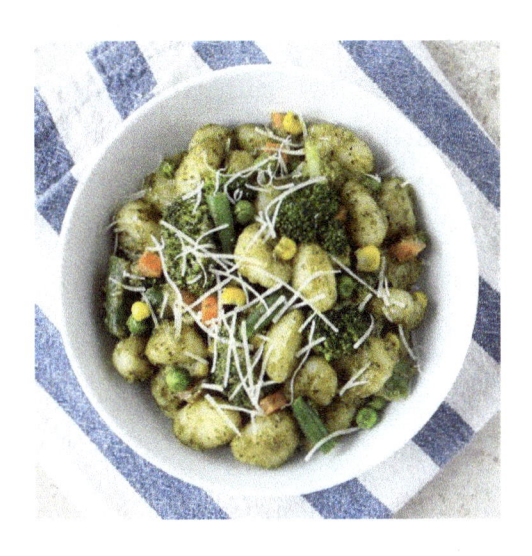

Ingredients

1 16-ounce package (450 g) of gnocchi
½ cup oil-dried tomatoes, chopped
¾ cup (80 ml) heavy cream
4 tablespoons pesto
½ teaspoon salt

Direction

Bring a pot of lightly salted water to the boil and cook the gnocchi according to the package instructions.

Heat the sun-dried tomato oil in a frying pan over a medium heat and fry the sun-dried tomatoes for a minute to release their aroma. Pour in the cream, cook for a minute (do not boil), remove from the heat and stir in the pesto. Season with salt.

Add the cooked and drained gnocchi to the sauce and stir until the gnocchi are coated with the sauce.

Serve warm. Top with grated Parmesan or vegetarian hard cheese, if desired.

9. Vegan Mushroom Risotto

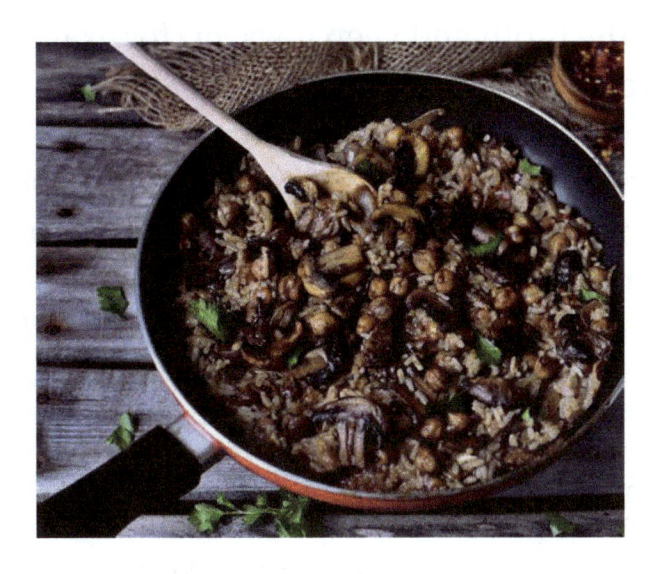

Ingredients

2 tbsp olive oil
2 cloves garlic
1 onion
3 cups vegetable broth (3 cups = 750 ml)
9 oz mushrooms (9oz = 250g or 2 cups)
½ cup risotto rice
2-3 tbsp nutritional yeast
2 tbsp parsley, fresh (or 1 tbsp dried parsle

Direction

Prepare the broth and keep it warm (for example, on the stove).
Quickly wash and slice the mushrooms.
Heat a large saucepan or frying pan and fry the mushrooms with a little oil until cooked through - about 5 minutes.
In the meantime, dice the onion and garlic. When the mushrooms are ready, set them aside and leave them for later.
In the same pan (without the mushrooms), fry the onions, adding more oil if necessary. Fry until soft.
Add the rice and fry for 2 minutes. Add the garlic and stir well. If using, add wine and cook until evaporated.
Now start pouring in the stock one ladle at a time. As soon as the liquid is almost gone, add another ladleful. This should give the risotto a nice creamy texture.
When the broth is used up and the rice is cooked, remove from the heat. Add the mushrooms and stir.
Top with vegan margarine, parsley and nutritional yeast. Cover with the lid.
After a couple of minutes the margarine should melt. Stir everything together.

10. Cheese Baked Rigatoni with Roasted Vegetables

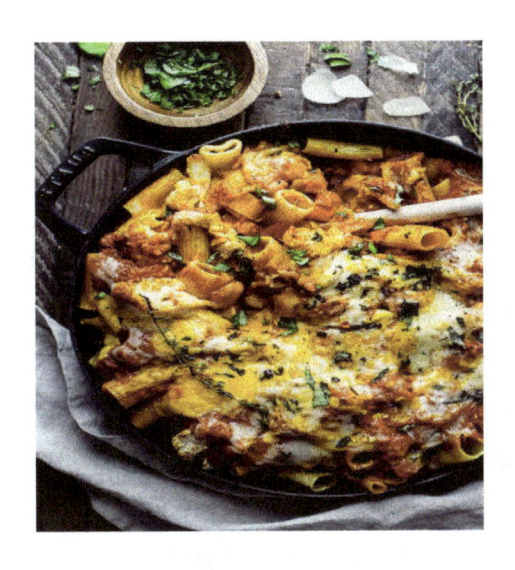

Ingredients

1 lb dry rigatoni pasta
3-4 cups marinara sauce
1-2 tablespoons oil
1 lb bag of small peppers
1 head of cauliflower
4-5 carrots
1/4 cup fresh basil, chopped
1 teaspoon oregano (dried or fresh)
1 cup grated cheddar cheese (divided)
1 cup grated gruyere cheese (divided)
1/2 cup grated Parmesan cheese
salt and black pepper

Direction

Preheat oven to 425F.
Prepare the vegetables: cut the cauliflower into petals. Remove the stem from the carrots, then cut them into sticks, cutting them lengthwise into quarters. Leave the small peppers whole (with stems). Roast the vegetables: place the vegetables on a baking tray and drizzle with oil. Stir and sprinkle with a pinch of salt and black pepper. Roast for 20 minutes (turning halfway through), then reduce the oven temperature to 325F and roast for a further 10 minutes.
Slice the vegetables: remove the roasted vegetables and cool slightly. Carefully remove the stems of the peppers. Cut the peppers and carrots into cubes. Chop the cauliflower if the pieces are too large, but leave the florets. Note: the roasted small peppers will be very soft, so you can easily remove the stems by gently pulling them out.
To make the pasta: While the vegetables are cooking, bring a large pot of water to the boil. Season the water with the pasta with plenty of salt (about 1-2 tablespoons). Cook the pasta as instructed on the box so that the pasta has an al dente texture. When draining the pasta, reserve 1/3 cup of water. Note: Al dente in Italian means "by the tooth" - the texture of the pasta should be bite-size and not too soft.

Mix the ingredients with the pasta: add 1-2 cups of marinara to the pot with the pasta and pasta water. Add 1/2 cup of cheddar cheese, 1/2 cup of gruyere cheese and 1/4 cup of parmesan cheese. Then add half of the roasted vegetables, chopped fresh basil and oregano.

Arrange in a baking dish. Add the remaining roasted vegetables and 1-2 cups of marinara, then sprinkle the remaining cheddar, gruyere and Parmesan cheeses on top.

Cover with foil or lid and bake at 350F for 20 minutes. For the last minute, bake on high to brown the cheese.

11. Pasta Arrabiata

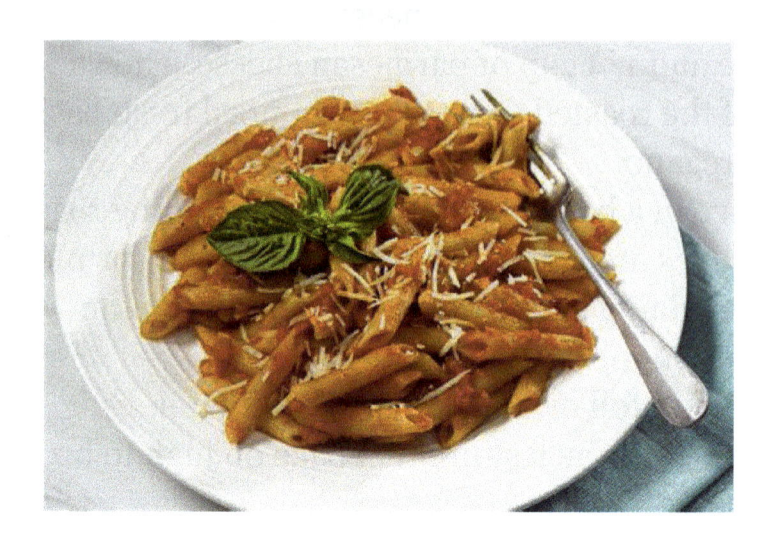

Ingredients

1 small aubergine
¼ tsp salt
8 oz wholegrain pasta (8oz = 250g)
¼ tsp paprika
1 medium onion
2 cloves garlic
2 medium tomato
¼ tsp sugar
3 tbsp olive oil
1 tsp tomato paste (also known as tomato concentrate – the thick stuff, often in a tube)
2 cups tomato juice (the drink) 2 cups = 500ml)
1 red chili pepper

2 tbsp almonds (roasted/smoked)

Direction

Cook the pasta as per packet instructions.
Wash and cut the aubergine and tomatoes into small pieces.
Heat up a pan with olive oil on a medium heat. Add the aubergine, and mix in the salt and paprika.
Dice the onion and garlic.
After a couple of minutes, add the onions and fry until soft. When they are, add the garlic and fry for another 30 seconds or so.
Add the tomato paste and let it fry for a couple of minutes more.
Add the tomato juice, the tomato pieces and the sugar.
Chop the chili pepper and throw that in there too.
Let it cook (bubbling) for another five minutes.
Crush the almonds.
Serve the pasta with the sauce, adding salt and pepper to taste. Garnish with the crushed almonds

12. Comforting Leek Risotto

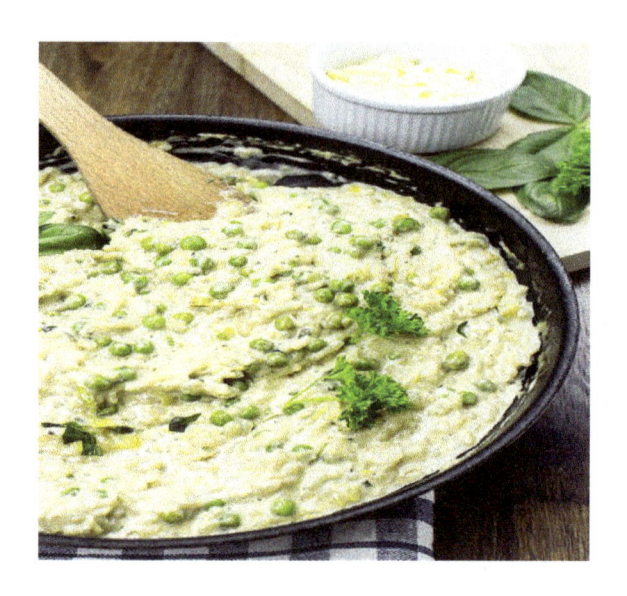

Ingredients

½ cup risotto rice
2-3 cups vegetable broth
½ leek
1 small onion
1 tbsp olive oil
1 cup peas, frozen
⅓ cup cream (⅓ cup = 100ml)
2.5 oz low fat cream cheese
2 tbsp soy sauce
2 tbsp Worcestershire sauce (vegetarian) (make sure to check for a no-fish version)
¼ tsp salt

¼ tsp pepper
1 tbsp basil, fresh
1 tbsp parsley, fresh
1 tbsp oregano, fresh (for all the herbs, dried or frozen are fine if fresh are unavailable)

Direction

Give the rice a quick rinse – we don't need this one too starchy.
Slice the leek and onion and fry in olive oil in a big pan on medium heat for about 5 Minutes.
Add the risotto rice and fry for another 2 minutes.
If using, throw in the white wine and stir until dissolved.
Add ¾ of the veggie broth. Let everything cook for about 20 minutes, or until the rice is ready. If it goes dry before the rice is ready, add more broth.
When the rice is ready, turn the heat off. Add the frozen peas, cream and cream cheese, soy sauce and Worcestershire sauce and basil, parsley and oregano. Give it a good stir making sure all is mixed together well.
Turn the heat back and cook on a med-high heat for another 5 minutes. This gives a chance for the sauce to become thick, and the flavours to fully come out. Add salt and pepper to taste. Just don't let it burn – stir occasionally!

Serve with a little cheddar sprinkled on the top for extra deliciousness.

13. Red Pesto Pasta

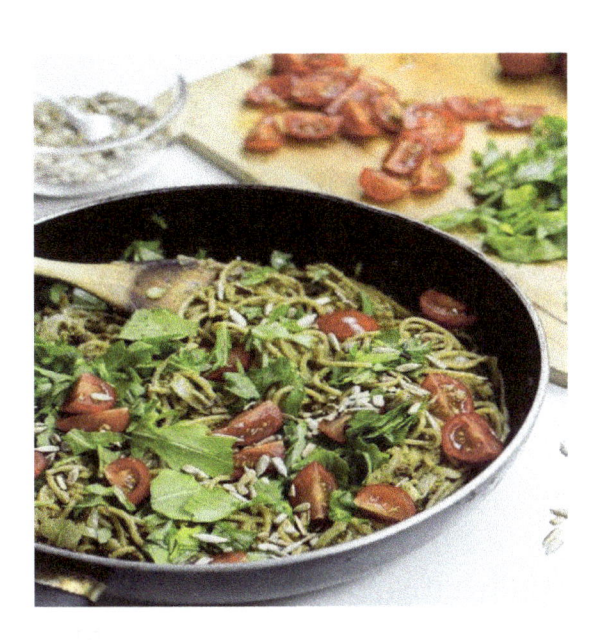

Ingredients

1 handful sunflower seeds (or use whatever seeds you have around)
7 oz pasta (wholegrain would be best)
1 onion
1 tbsp olive oil
3-4 tbsp red pesto (See notes below to make your own!)
1 handful spinach (1 handful = 50g, arugula also works)
1 handful cherry tomatoes

Direction

Boil that pasta o'yours.
Dice the onion and fry it with olive oil in a pan on medium heat.
While that's cooking put the seeds in a frying pan and fry without oil. They'll only take a minute or two so don't let them burn!
Drain the cooked pasta then add it into the pan, mix in red pesto, spinach/arugula and a good handful of diced cherry tomatoes.
Add a few splashes of water if you want it a bit creamier.
Depending on what you want add rennet-free cheddar cheese for taste, or leave it out for a vegan version.
For serving add a couple more cherry tomatoes as a garnish, and sprinkle over the sunflower seeds.

14. Vegetarian Zucchini

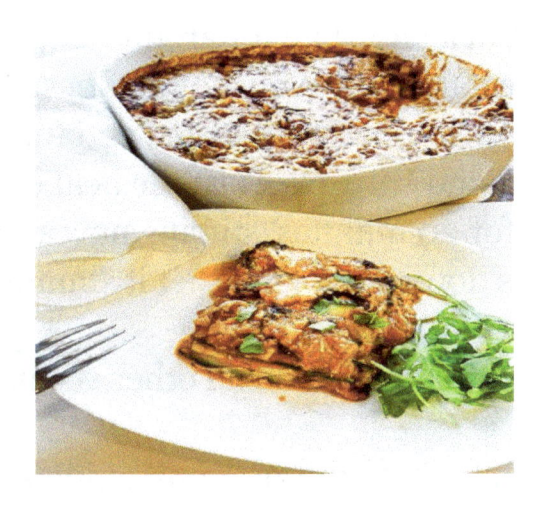

Ingredients

½ cup spelt grains, ground (usually referred to as 'cracked' and/or 'cracked freekeh')
2 cups vegetable broth
2 medium zucchini
1 tbsp olive oil
1 onion
Lasagna sheets
1 can tomato passata
2 tbsp tomato paste
1 cup bechamel sauce (you can make your own if you like)
salt and pepper to taste
1 tbsp basil, dried (you can also use fresh basil)
3.5 oz cheddar cheese

Direction

Fry the spelt in a large pan for around 2-3 minutes on a medium heat (no oil). Watch out it doesn't burn! Just as it starts to release its aroma and turn brown, add the stock and stir well. Turn the heat off and let the spelt sit for 20 minutes, stirring now and then. If the pan cools down completely, let it simmer on a low heat instead.

Dice the zucchini, onion and all other veg into tiny pieces.

After 20 minutes, add the zucchini, onion and any other veg into the spelt, along with the tomato puree and tomato paste.

Also add salt, pepper and basil. Taste test, and if the tomato wasn't particularly sweet, add a tsp sugar to offset it. Let it all simmer on a low-medium heat for around 10 mins.

Prep time next: Add ⅓ of the spelt/veg mix to an oven tray. Layer lasagna sheets over it, and on top of that add ⅓ bechamel sauce, using a spoon to spread it over the sheets . Add the next ⅓ spelt/veg mix, more lasagna sheets and another ⅓ bechamel sauce. Finally add the rest of the veg mix and another layer of bechamel sauce (no more lasagna sheets). On the top layer, sprinkle the grated cheese. Ready!

Into the oven for 35 minutes on 200°C/390°F, or until a deep golden brown. Best lasagna ever.

15. Crispy Tortilla Pizza

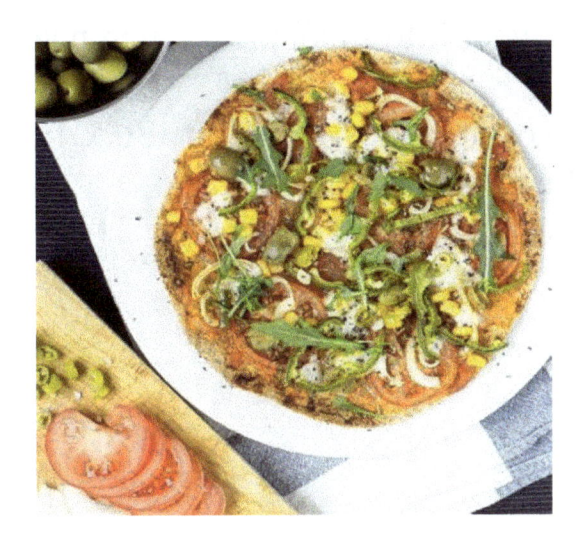

Ingredients

4 tortillas (whole wheat ideally)
1 tomato puree
1 ball mozzarella cheese (feta or most other cheeses work fine)
1 handful olives
1 white or red onion
1 chilli / jalapeño
4 small tomato
½ bell pepper, red (your fave colour)
½ cup basil, fresh (dried is fine but use much less)

Direction

Spread the tomato puree over each tortilla.

Lob on the basil.

Slice the cheese into thin layers and add to tortillas.

Chop the veggies into small pieces then place evenly on tortillas

Cook in the oven for 10-15 mins at 180°C (360°F) – don't let the tortillas burn!

Munch.

16. Lemon Pappardelle

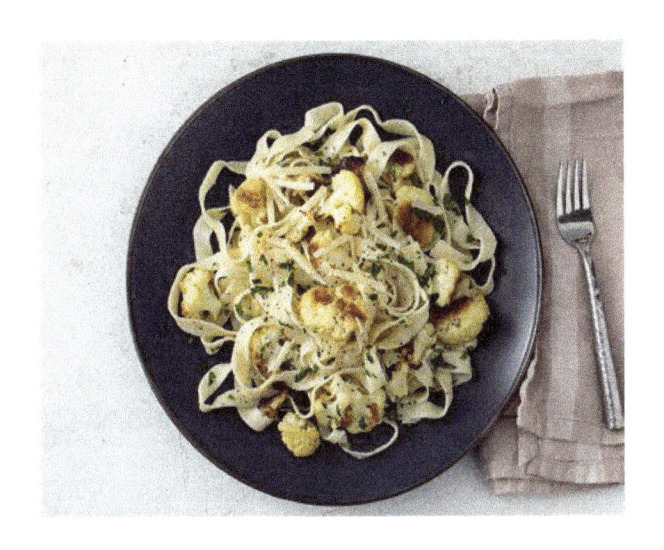

Ingredients

200 g fresh pappardelle pasta (egg free if vegan)
1 tbsp olive oil
2 medium unwaxed lemons (zest and juice)
2 tbsp pine nuts (toasted)
For basil and kale pesto:
1 large bunch of fresh basil (plus extra few leaves to decorate)
2 tsp kale powder
2 tbsp olive oil (extra virgin)
2 tbsp white wine vinegar
2 tbsp natural yogurt (dairy free)
1 tsp dijon mustard (optional)
salt and pepper to taste

Direction

Bring a large sauce pan of water to boil and cook fresh pappardelle for 4 minutes.

In a meantime, make basil and kale pesto. Place all the ingredients into food processor and blitz until well combined. Add a spoon of water if you prefer your pesto a bit less thick.

Drain cooked pasta, drizzle with olive oil. Pour the pesto over pasta, add zest and juice of lemon, and toss all together. Top with toasted pine nuts and fresh basil leaves.

17. Smoky Baked Eggs with Ricotta and Beans

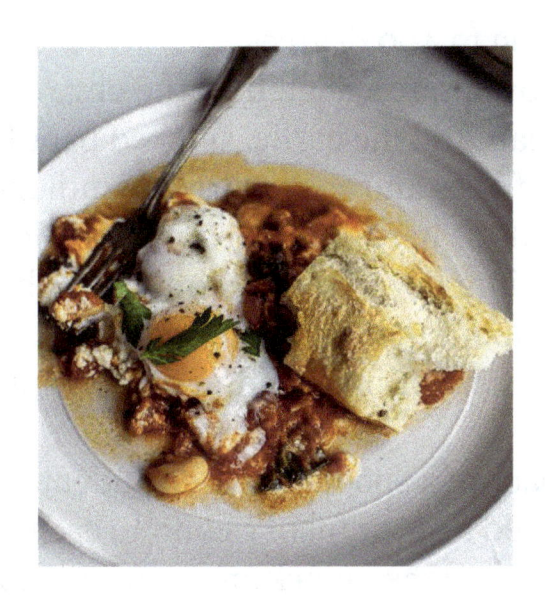

Ingredients

1/4 Cup olive oil
2 Cloves garlic, minced
3/4 Teaspoon smoked paprika
1/4 Teaspoon red pepper flakes
1 (15 ounce) Can cannellini beans, drained and rinsed
1 (28 ounce) Can crushed tomatoes
Handful of fresh baby spinach (optional)
1 1/2 Cups ricotta
6 Eggs
Salt and pepper, to taste
Fresh herbs, roughly chopped
Crusty bread, for serving

Direction

Pre heat oven to 400 degrees.
In a large, oven safe skillet, heat the olive oil over medium heat. Add the garlic, smoked paprika, and red pepper flakes and cook, stirring, until fragrant; 1 minute. Add the beans and the tomatoes, lower the heat to medium low, and cook until sauce has thickened; about 15 minutes. Season with salt and pepper to taste. Stir in a handful of baby spinach, if using.
With the back of a spoon, make six indentations in the sauce, add a spoonful of ricotta to each indentation, and then crack an egg over the ricotta. Transfer the skillet to the oven and bake until egg whites are set but yolks are still runny (the eggs will continue to cook a bit in the pan) about 12-15 minutes.
Garnish with your favorite fresh herbs and serve with warm crusty bread.

18. Creamy Broccoli Pasta

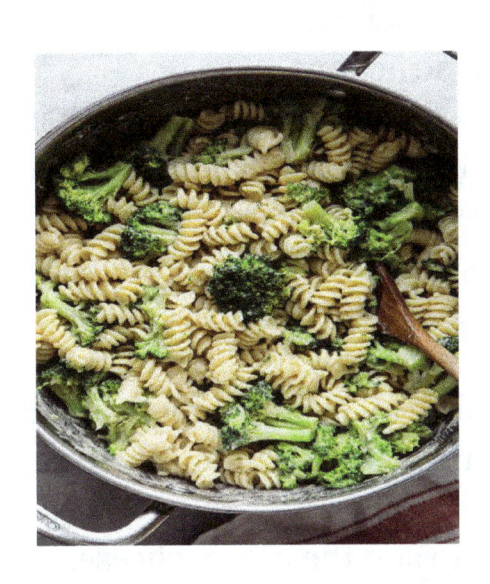

Ingredients

7 oz pasta (e.g. tagliatelle or linguine)
2 tbsp olive oil
2 cups broccoli (frozen is fine too)
1 onion
2 cloves garlic
½ cup vegetable broth
4 oz cream cheese
1 tsp honey
1 tsp lemon juice
salt and pepper to taste
1 tsp chili flakes

Direction

Bring water to a boil and cook the pasta according to the package instructions.

If you're using frozen broccoli, throw it in a pan right away with 3 tbsp of olive oil and cover with a lid – the broccoli thaws more quickly.

If using fresh, wash and cut the fresh broccoli into small florets. Next, peel and dice the onion; same with the cloves of garlic.

Heat up the olive oil in a pan, then add the broccoli, onion and garlic. On medium heat let everything simmer for 5 minutes.

Now it's time to add the cream cheese.

Now slowly pour in the vegetable broth. NOTE: If you think the mixture is getting watery, stop pouring!

Once ready, drain the pasta in a sieve. Now add them to the broccoli cream mix. Cook on medium heat for another 5 minutes

Add salt, pepper and a few chili flakes to taste. To give it another kick, give a few splashes of lemon juice and a tsp of honey to the mix.

19. Italian Summer Vegetable Casserole

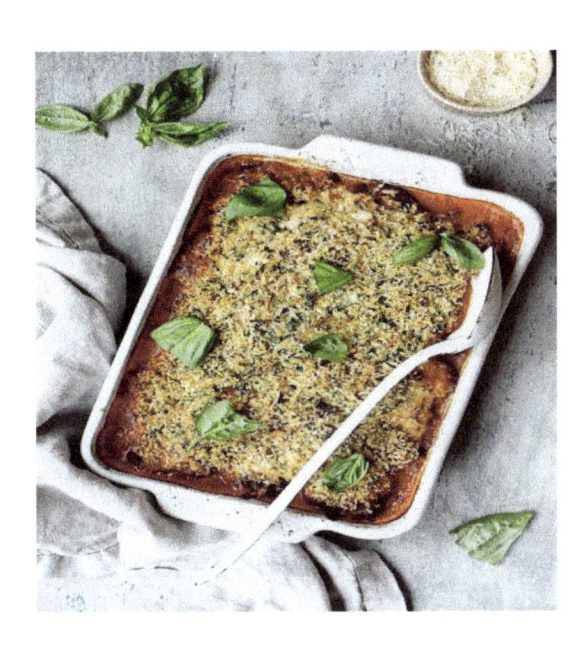

Ingredients

1 medium sized aubergine, cut into ¼ inch thick slices
2 small to medium yellow squash, sliced into ¼ inch thick slices
2 medium sized courgettes, cut into ¼ inch thick slices
1 large red pepper, seedless, stemless and cored, cut into approximately 12 long strips
1 large yellow pepper, seedless, stemless and cored, cut into approximately 12 long strips
¼ cup olive oil and 2 tablespoons
salt and freshly ground black pepper to taste

Cooking spray
1 jar (24 ounces) of marinara sauce such as Bertolli olive oil and garlic
2 large sprigs of fresh basil, leaves torn
3 cups shredded Mozzarella cheese
1 cup freshly grated Parmesan cheese
½ cup panko
2 tablespoons chopped fresh parsley

Direction

Preheat the grill to medium-high. Lightly brush the vegetables with ¼ cup olive oil. Place the vegetables on the grill and reduce the heat to medium. Grill the vegetables until nicely charred and slightly softened, except for the aubergines. Roast the aubergines until they are easy to pierce with a knife.
Preheat oven to 375 degrees. Spray a 13 x 9 inch baking dish with cooking spray.
Spread the bottom of the prepared baking dish with about ½ cup of marinara sauce.
Place the zucchini on top of the sauce to cover the bottom, then top with ½ cup of marinara and sprinkle with about ½ cup of mozzarella, sprinkle with parmesan cheese and some torn basil. Place the red peppers on top.
Top with the remaining zucchini and yellow squash, ½ cup of sauce, ½ cup of Mozzarella, more Parmesan and more torn basil.

Place the yellow peppers on top, then the aubergine. Pour the remaining marinara sauce over the roast. Top with the remaining Mozzarella and more Parmesan, leaving about ¼ cup of the dressing.

In a small bowl, mix together the remaining ¼ cup Parmesan, panko, parsley and the remaining 2 tablespoons olive oil. Sprinkle over the top of the roast.

Bake for 45 minutes or until the top is bubbling and lightly browned.

20. Creamy Avocado Pasta

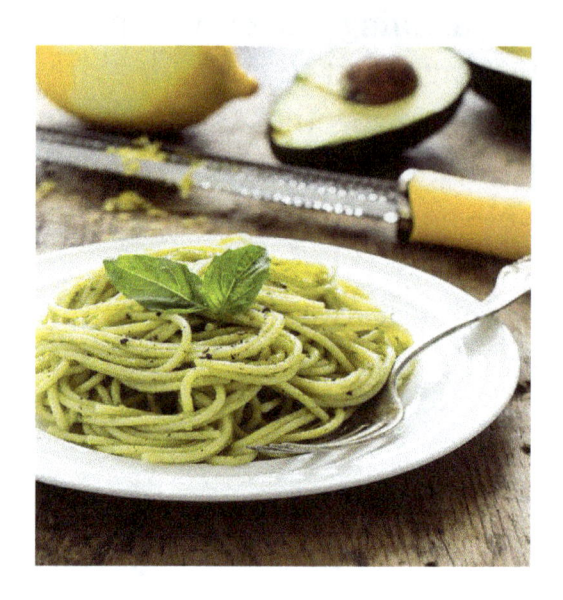

Ingredients

5 oz whole grain pasta
1 cup cherry tomatoes
¼ cup basil, fresh (dry basil will do too, but use less)
1 large avocado
2-3 tbsp lemon juice
1-2 tbsp soy sauce
1 tbsp olive oil
1 clove garlic
salt to taste
Add a few tbsps of water, if too thick.

Direction

Bring water to boil and chuck in pasta.
Use pasta cooking time to prepare the avocado sauce:
Mash the avocado flesh with a fork in a bowl until its creamy (if you have a food processor, use that)
Add olive oil, lemon juice and soy sauce to the mashed avocado
Cut the basil leaves and add them to the bowl
Grate the garlic and ginger and add them too. Remember, ginger is optional. Unless you're born that way
If the mix is too thick then add some tablespoons of water
Drain the pasta and place it back in the pot. Add the avocado sauce and stir nicely
Halve the cherry tomatoes and throw in with pasta
Sprinkle with sesame seeds if you have them to hand and season with a bit of salt.

21. Brown Rice Risotto with Butternut Squash & Mushrooms

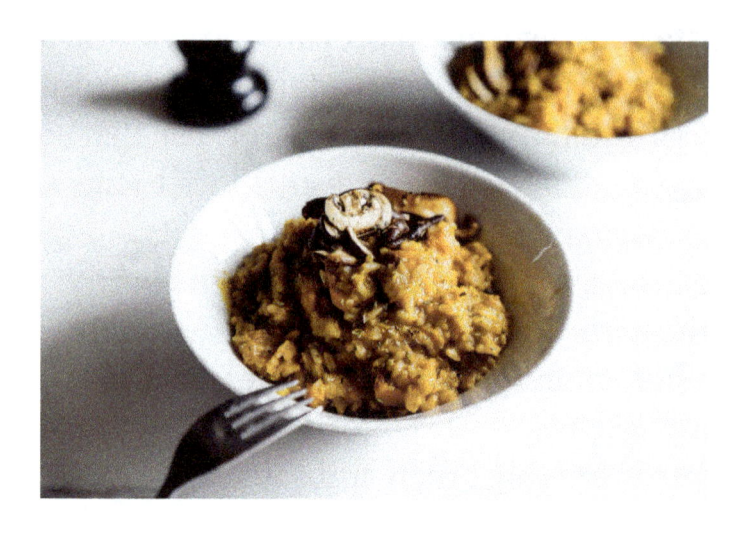

Ingredients

1 1/2 Tbsp. avocado oil, divided (or whatever kid of oil you prefer)
3/4 lb. butternut squash, cubed into 1 cm cubes
8 oz. mushrooms, quartered
1 small onion, diced
1 tsp. minced garlic
1 cup sprouted short grain brown rice*
1/2 cup dry white wine (sauvignon blanc works great)
6 cups broth (either chicken or vegetable)
5 oz. fresh baby spinach
2 Tbsp. freshly chopped sage
1/8 tsp. nutmeg
1/4 cup grated parmesan

1/4 cup toasted walnuts, crushed*
salt and pepper to taste

Direction

Preheat oven to 425° F (218° C).
Rub butternut squash with 1/2 T oil and sprinkle with salt and pepper on a large baking sheet. Place in oven and roast for about 10 minutes.
After squash have baked for 10 minutes, add mushrooms to same pan as squash (or a separate pan if there isn't room), rub with 1/2 T oil and place pan back in oven for about 15 minutes until squash and mushrooms are fully cooked.
Heat 1/2 Tbsp. oil in a large saucepan over medium heat. Add onion and sauté for 2-3 minutes to soften. Add garlic and cook for another minute.
Add rice to pan with onion and garlic and stir for 2-3 minutes. Add white wine to rice and stir until mostly absorbed.
Ladle 1/2 cup broth into pan with rice and stir until mostly absorbed. Continue adding broth half a cup at a time, stirring continuously. Repeat adding more broth every few minutes when rice has absorbed most of liquid (takes 20-30 minutes total).
Add spinach and sage to rice and stir 1 minute until spinach is wilted.

Remove from heat and add mushrooms, butternut squash, toasted walnuts, nutmeg, and parmesan. Season with salt and pepper and serve immediately.

22. Spaghetti cacio e pepe

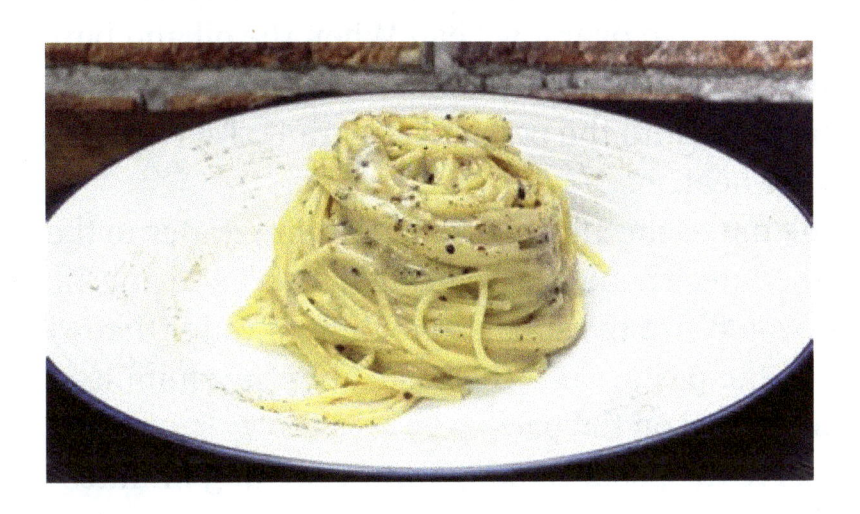

Ingredients

9 oz (250g) spaghetti
5 oz (135g) Pecorino cheese, aged Pecorino Toscano or Pecorino Romano cheese
1/2 cup pasta cooking water it's good to have more on hand
1 tablespoon butter
1 tablespoon olive oil
1-2 teaspoons freshly ground black pepper

Direction
Prepare all the ingredients: grate the cheese on the microplane zester (it's the best) or on the smallest holes of a box grater, grind the pepper.

Set aside.

Toast the pepper: Heat the olive oil and butter in a big frying pan over low heat. When the oil and butter are hot, add the pepper. Cook, stirring, for about a minute or until the pepper is fragrant. Take the pan off the heat.

Cook the pasta: In a medium pot bring water to the boil. Water should be well-salted, don't add any oil to the water, use the smallest amount of water that will cover the pasta. Cook the pasta about 1-2 minutes less than it says on the package.

Reserve the pasta cooking water: About 3 minutes before the end of the cooking time reserve about 1 cup of pasta cooking water. We will need only 1/2 cup for this recipe but it's always good to have more on hand if you need to dilute the sauce.

Add the 1/2 cup of the water to the pan and whisk intensively to combine it with butter and olive oil. Set aside. Reserve the remaining pasta cooking water. Add the cooked pasta to the pan and toss it with the sauce. Let stand for about a minute or two, letting it cool slightly before adding the cheese.

Add the cheese and stir very intensively with kitchen tongs or two forks until the cheese is melted, creamy, and creates a smooth silky sauce. You can put the pan on the burner while you do this and heat it over very low heat to help melt the cheese. If the cheese doesn't melt easily add some more reserved pasta cooking water. Heat the sauce gently over low heat until all the cheese is melted.

Taste the pasta and season with more pepper if necessary.

23. Italian Tortellini Spinach Soup

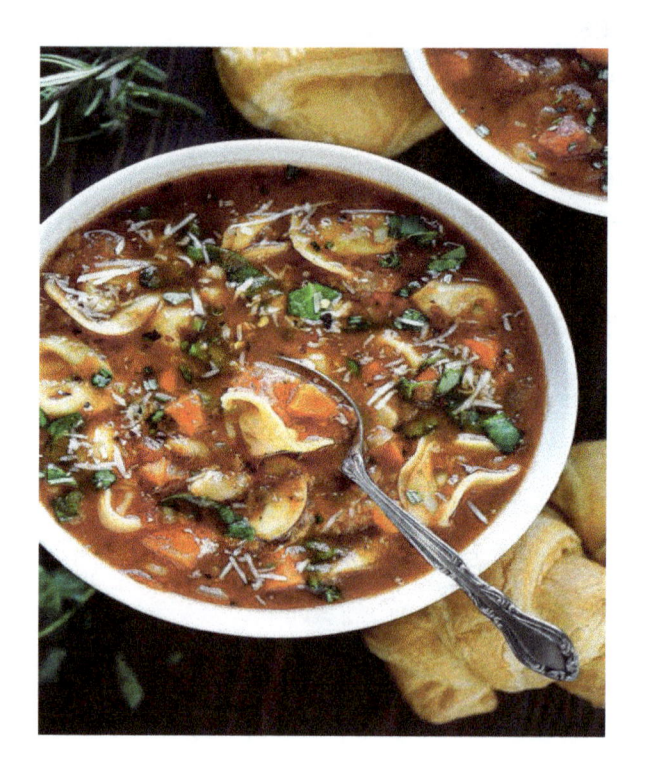

Ingredients

1 tsp olive oil
1 large clove garlic minced
4 cups chicken broth
2 cups low sodium chicken broth*
1 14- oz can fire-roasted tomatoes
1/2 tsp Italian seasoning
1/2 tsp dried basil
1 12- oz package cheese tortellini
6- oz bag fresh baby spinach

Fresh parmesan cheese to serve optional

Direction

Place large soup pot over medium heat. Add 1 tsp olive oil to pot. Once oil is warm, add garlic and sauté for 30sec-1 min, or until fragrant.
Add broth, tomatoes, and seasonings. Bring to a simmer and continue to simmer for 5 minutes.
Add in dried packaged tortellini and bring to a gentle boil. Cook for 10 minutes (do not fully cook the tortellini yet, you want it al-dente).
Reduce to a simmer and add in spinach. Simmer for 5 minutes or until spinach is wilted and tortellini is completely cooked.
Divide into 4 bowls and top with freshly shredded parmesan cheese.

24. Tomato Mozzarella Bread

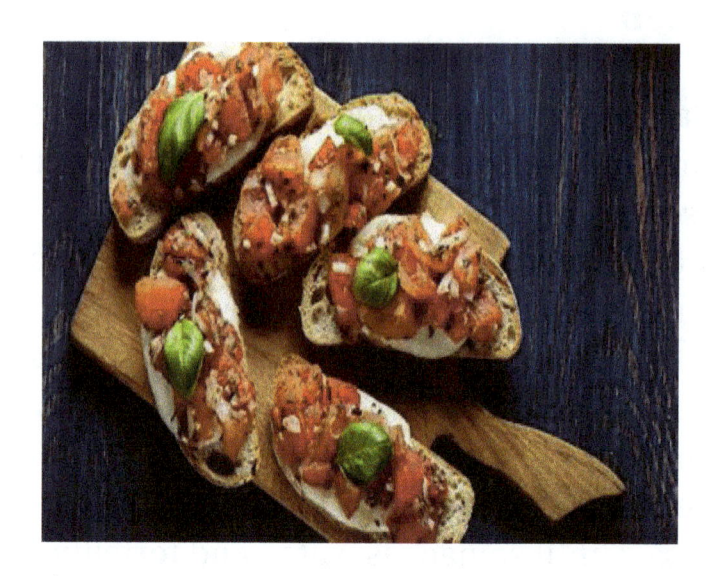

Ingredients

½ cup cherry tomatoes (or swap ½ cup cherry tomatoes for 1 large tomato. Dave prefers the former, Hauke the latter. Choose your side!)
1 ball low fat mozzarella cheese (1 ball = ca. 125g/4.5oz)
¼ cup basil, fresh fresh
1 tbsp olive oil
1 tbsp balsamic vinegar
salt and pepper to taste
2-3 slices bread (whole wheat; or rustic/farm bread)

Direction

Preheat oven to 180°C/360°F.
Slice the tomatoes to about 1/4 cm thick and the cheese a little thinner.
Spread a little olive oil on the bread
Layer the mozzarella and then the tomatoes on the bread.
Chop and add basil, salt and pepper.
Bung in oven for 5 mins or so, or until golden brown with melted cheese.
Put the vinegar on last for the fullest flavour.

25. Caprese Salad

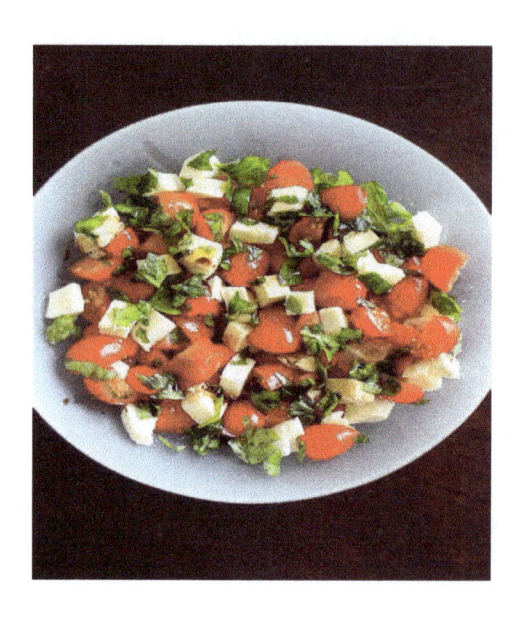

Ingredients

3 large ripe tomatoes sliced into ¼ inch thickness
12 ounces (350g) fresh mozzarella cheese sliced into ¼ inch thickness
2 tablespoons extra virgin olive oil
½ teaspoon sea salt flakes
¼ teaspoon ground black pepper
2 tablespoons balsamic reduction/glaze optional

Direction

Layer the tomato and mozzarella slices in a serving platter alternating between the two.

Tuck in fresh basil leaves between every slice of tomato and mozzarella. Arrange the ingredients so you're able to see the layers in the platter. Drizzle with olive oil.

Season with salt, pepper, and drizzle with balsamic reduction/glaze if using.

26. Italian Sauteed Swiss Chard

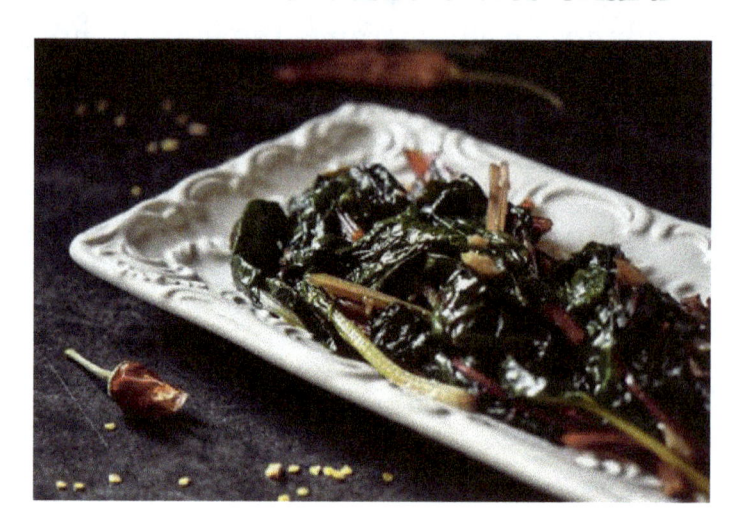

Ingredients

1 bunch Swiss chard fresh or rainbow chard
2 tablespoons olive oil
2-3 cloves garlic coarsely chopped
pinch crushed red pepper or more-according to taste
1-2 tablespoons water optional
salt and pepper to taste
olive oil for drizzling
Parmesan cheese shavings optional

Direction

Set a large pot of salted water to boil.
Meanwhile, properly rinse the chard to remove dirt and sand.
Trim off the ends. Cut off the ribs from the leafy part.

Once the water has started boiling, throw in the ribs. Boil for 3-5 minutes or until beginning to soften.
Add the green leaves and continue to boil for approximately 1-2 minutes.
Drain thoroughly in a colander
Add the olive oil, the chopped garlic and a pinch of red pepper flakes (if using) to a large skillet.
Turn the heat on to medium and sauté for 2 to 3 minutes.
Once the garlic begins to turn a light golden brown, remove from heat and add the parboiled Swiss chard. Watch for splattering.
Use tongs to turn it over to properly coat it with the garlic-infused oil.
Place the pan back on the heat, and season with salt and pepper according to taste.
Cover the skillet and allow it to cook for up to 5 minutes or until tender but still a little crisp. If necessary add a few tablespoons of water.
Taste and adjust for seasonings.
Place on serving dish and drizzle with olive oil and shavings of Parmesan cheese.

27. The Bruschetta

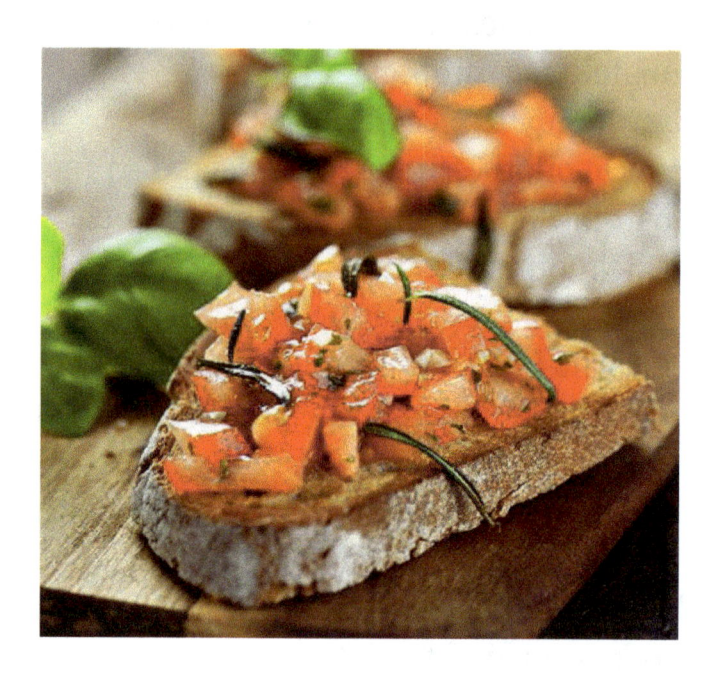

Ingredients

1 Baguette, sliced on an angle
5 Roma tomatoes, diced
2 Cloves garlic, smashed
Juice from 1 Lemon
Goat Cheese
Fresh Basil, chiffonade
Olive oil
Pinch of salt and pepper

Direction

Pre heat the oven to 400 degrees.
Slice the baguette on an angle and brush each piece with olive oil. On a baking sheet, toast the bread slices in the oven until golden brown; about 15 minutes.
Make the tomato mixture. In a large bowl, toss the chopped tomatoes, salt and pepper, and lemon together. Set aside.
When the breads are golden brown, remove them from the oven and rub them with the garlic cloves. Spread the goat cheese on each toast and top with the tomato mixture and fresh basil.

28. Verza Stufata

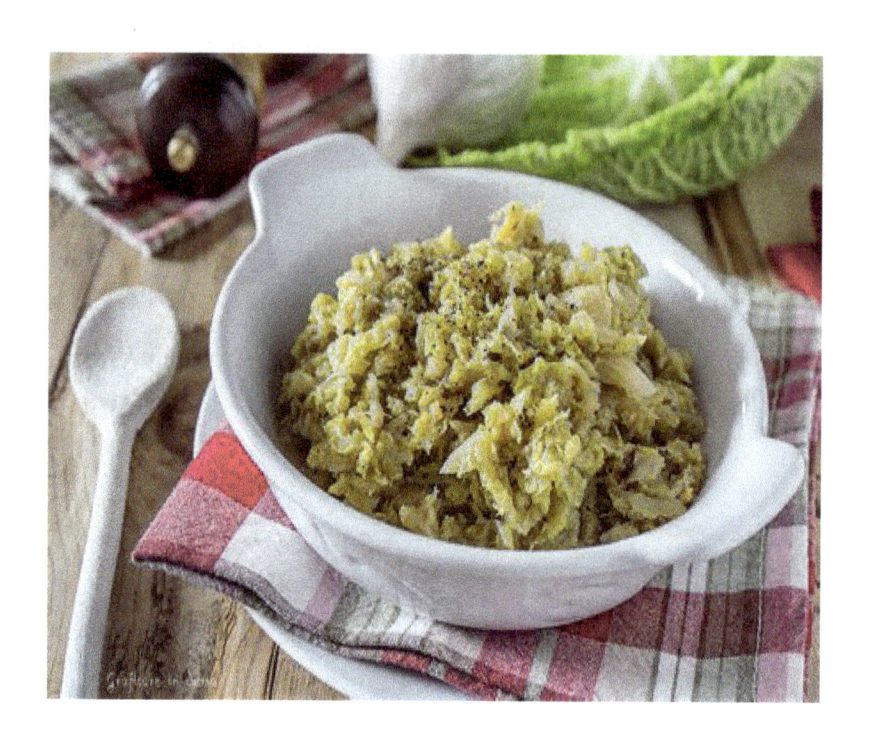

Ingredients

3 tablespoons olive oil
1 large garlic clove chopped small
1 savoy cabbage washed and patted dry
200 ml vegetable stock (1 cup) or beef/chicken stock
½ teaspoon salt to taste
⅛ teaspoon black pepper freshly ground
olive oil from drizzling (optional)

Direction

Prepare the cabbage by slicing down the middle, cutting away the tough central core, the slicing the leaves into thin 1 inch strips.

In a large saucepan with a lid, heat the oil with garlic on low heat till the garlic softens.

Add sliced cabbage, turn the heat to medium and sauté for a couple of minutes in the garlic oil.

Stir in a third of the stock, then turn the heat back down to low, cover and leave to simmer for 30 minutes, lifting the lid occasionally to stir, and adding more stock gradually.

Remove from the heat, and serve warm with a drizzle of olive oil over the top and a grating of cheese.

29. Italian Vegetarian Stuffed Mushrooms

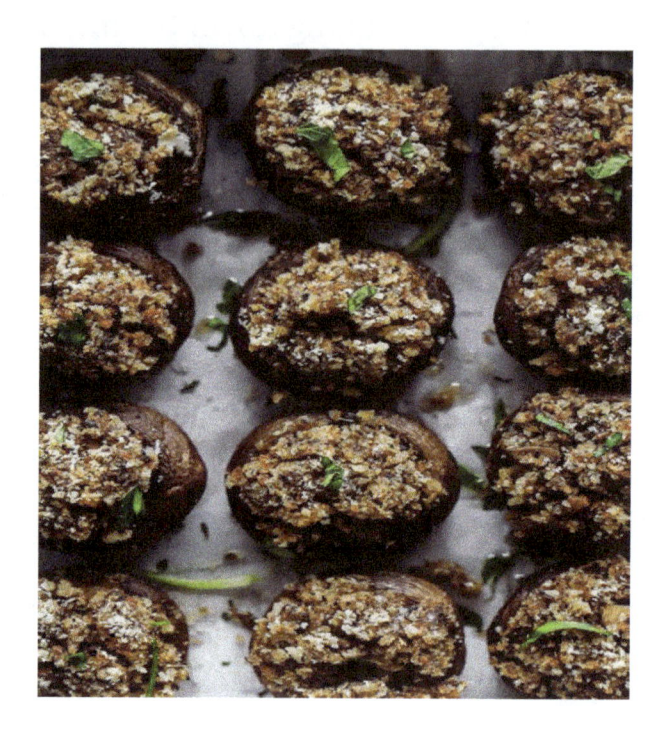

Ingredients

12 whole mushrooms about 2 inches in diameter (I used small portobello mushrooms)
1/4 cup extra-virgin olive oil divided
1/4 cup shallots finely diced (or onion)
2 cloves garlic minced
3 tablespoons fresh parsley finely chopped, plus more for garnish
1/2 cup breadcrumbs
1/4 cup parmesan cheese fresh grated, see notes

1/2 teaspoon dried oregano or 1 teaspoon finely chopped fresh
kosher salt to taste
black pepper to taste

Direction

Gently wipe off any excess dirt from the mushrooms with a clean kitchen or paper towel. Don't wash them with water, as this will affect their texture.
Remove the stems from the mushrooms. Cut off and discard the tough ends. Finely chop the stems.
Heat a skillet (I used nonstick) over medium heat. Add 2 tablespoons olive oil.
Add the shallots, garlic, mushrooms, and parsley to the skillet with a pinch of salt. Cook until ingredients are softened, stirring occasionally, about 5-7 minutes.
In a medium bowl, mix the sautéed mushroom mixture with the breadcrumbs, parmesan cheese, oregano, and salt + pepper to taste.
Place the mushrooms in a baking dish. Stuff them with the mixture, pressing down to get as much in as possible. Use ALL the stuffing- some of it may not fit and fall off the sides, this is OK!
Drizzle the remaining two tablespoons olive oil on top of the stuffed mushrooms.
Cover the baking sheet with foil. (At this point, you can refrigerate the mushrooms for up to a day to be baked later.)

Bake at 375 degrees for 20 minutes. Remove foil and bake 10-15 more minutes, until mushrooms are golden and bubbling.

30. Homemade Basil Pesto

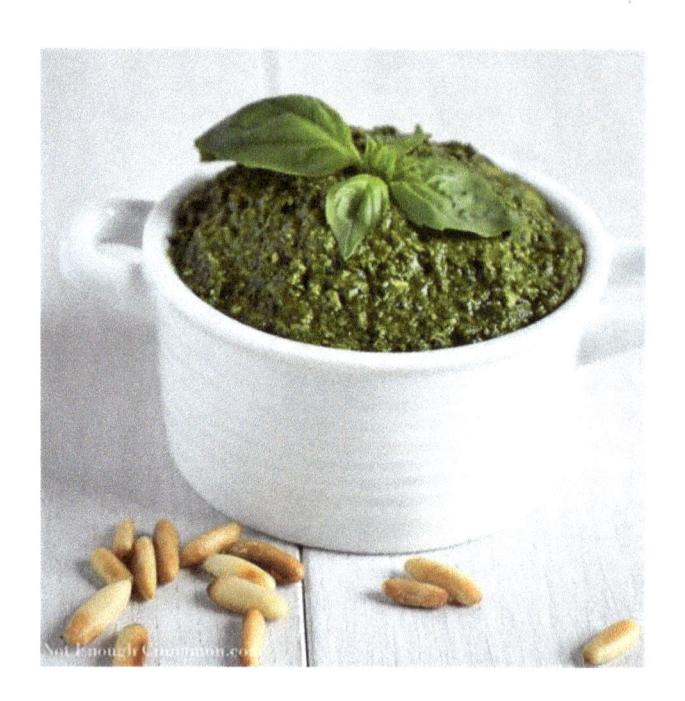

Ingredients

1 cup basil, fresh
¼ cup vegetarian parmesan, grated (make sure to use a non-animal rennet version if you're vegetarian. ¼ cup = ca. 25g)
3 tbsp walnuts
1 clove garlic
¾ tsp salt
½ tsp pepper
5 tbsp olive oil

Direction

Chop the basil leaves and nuts and place in a large glass.
Grate the garlic and cheese (if using) and add to the mixture, along with the salt and pepper.
Add the oil and mix well with a spoon. Alternatively you can use a hand blender or food processor to mix everything together.
If necessary, transfer to a smaller glass for storing, and pour on a little more oil to seal the pesto.
Cover in cling wrap and it should keep for up to two weeks in the fridge.

31. Eggplant Rollatini

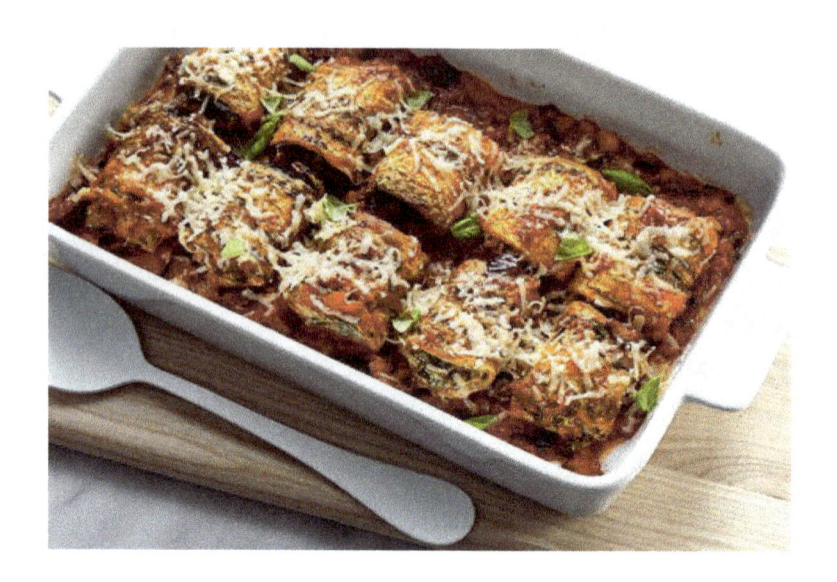

Ingredients

1 large eggplant
1 tablespoon salt
SAUCE:
1 small onion, chopped
1/4 cup olive oil
2 garlic cloves, minced
1 can (15 ounces) tomato sauce
1 can (14-1/2 ounces) diced tomatoes
1/2 cup chicken broth
1/4 cup tomato paste
2 tablespoons minced fresh parsley
2 teaspoons sugar

1/2 teaspoon salt
1/2 teaspoon dried basil
1/4 teaspoon pepper
1/8 teaspoon crushed red pepper flakes

Directions

Peel and slice eggplant lengthwise into fifteen 1/8-in.-thick slices. Place in a colander over a plate; sprinkle with salt and toss. Let stand 30 minutes.
Meanwhile, for sauce, in a large saucepan, saute onion in oil. Add garlic; cook 1 minute longer. Stir in remaining sauce ingredients. Bring to a boil. Reduce heat; simmer, uncovered, until flavors are blended, stirring occasionally, 20-25 minutes. Rinse and drain eggplant.
In a large bowl, combine filling ingredients; set aside. Place eggs in a shallow bowl. In another shallow bowl, combine bread crumbs, 1/2 cup Parmesan cheese, garlic, parsley, salt and pepper. Dip eggplant in eggs, then bread crumb mixture.
In an electric skillet or deep skillet, heat 1/2 in. of oil to 375°. Fry eggplant in batches until golden brown, 2-3 minutes on each side. Drain on paper towels.

Preheat oven to 375°. Spoon 1 cup sauce into an ungreased 13x9-in. baking dish. Spread 2 rounded tablespoons filling over each eggplant slice. Carefully roll up and place seam side down in baking dish. Spoon remaining sauce over roll-ups. Sprinkle with remaining Parmesan cheese. Cover and bake until bubbly, 30-35 minutes.

32. Homemade Ravioli

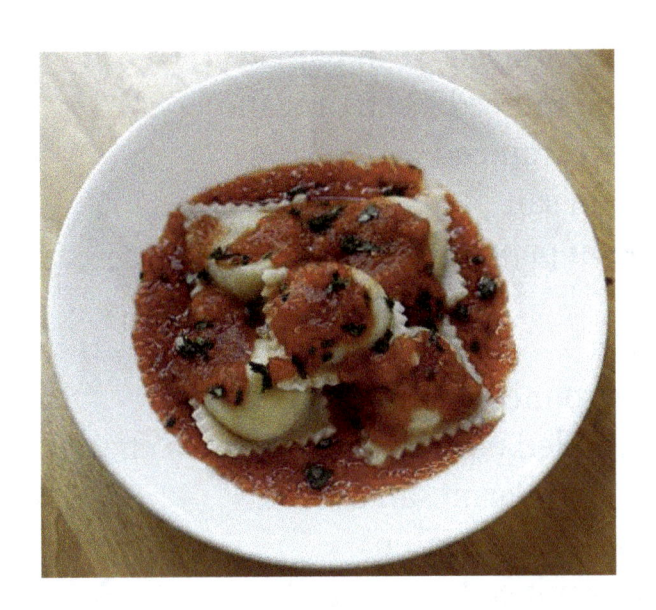

Ingredients

5 to 5-1/2 cups all-purpose flour
6 large eggs
1/2 cup water
1 tablespoon olive oil
SAUCE:
1 can (28 ounces) crushed tomatoes
1-1/2 cups tomato puree
1/2 cup grated Parmesan cheese
1/3 cup water
1/3 cup tomato paste

3 tablespoons sugar
2 tablespoons minced fresh basil
1 tablespoon minced fresh parsley
1 tablespoon minced fresh oregano
1 garlic clove, minced
1/2 teaspoon salt
1/4 teaspoon pepper

FILLING:
1 carton (15 ounces) ricotta cheese
2 cups shredded part-skim mozzarella cheese
1/3 cup grated Parmesan cheese
1 large egg, lightly beaten
2 teaspoons minced fresh basil
1 teaspoon minced fresh parsley
1 teaspoon minced fresh oregano
1/4 teaspoon garlic powder
1/8 teaspoon salt
1/8 teaspoon pepper

Directions

Place 5 cups flour in a large bowl. Make a well in the center. Beat the eggs, water and oil; pour into well. Stir together, forming a ball. Turn onto a floured surface; knead until smooth and elastic, about 4-6 minutes, adding remaining flour if necessary to keep dough from sticking. Cover and let rest for 30 minutes.

Meanwhile, in a Dutch oven, combine sauce ingredients. Bring to a boil. Reduce heat; cover and simmer for 1 hour, stirring occasionally.

In a large bowl, combine filling ingredients. Cover and refrigerate until ready to use.

Divide pasta dough into fourths; roll 1 portion to 1/16-in. thickness. (Keep pasta covered until ready to use.) Working quickly, place rounded teaspoonfuls of filling 1 in. apart over half of pasta sheet. Fold sheet over; press down to seal. Cut into squares with a pastry wheel. Repeat with remaining dough and filling.

Bring a soup kettle of salted water to a boil. Add ravioli. Reduce heat to a gentle simmer; cook until ravioli float to the top and are tender, 1-2 minutes. Drain. Spoon sauce over ravioli.

33. Linguine with Fresh Tomatoes

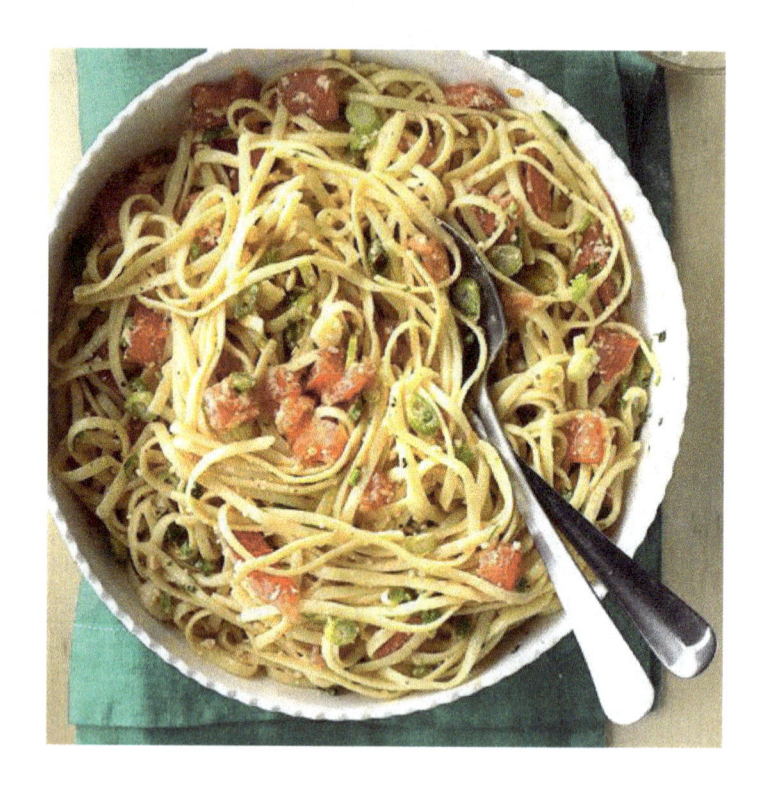

Ingredients

8 ounces uncooked linguine
3 medium tomatoes, chopped
6 green onions, sliced
1/2 cup grated Parmesan cheese
1/4 cup minced fresh basil or 4 teaspoons dried basil
2 garlic cloves, minced
1 teaspoon salt
1/2 teaspoon pepper
3 tablespoons butter

Directions

Cook linguine according to package directions. Meanwhile, place all remaining ingredients except butter in a large bowl.
Drain linguine; toss with butter. Add to tomato mixture and toss to combine.

34. Cherry Tomato & Basil Focaccia

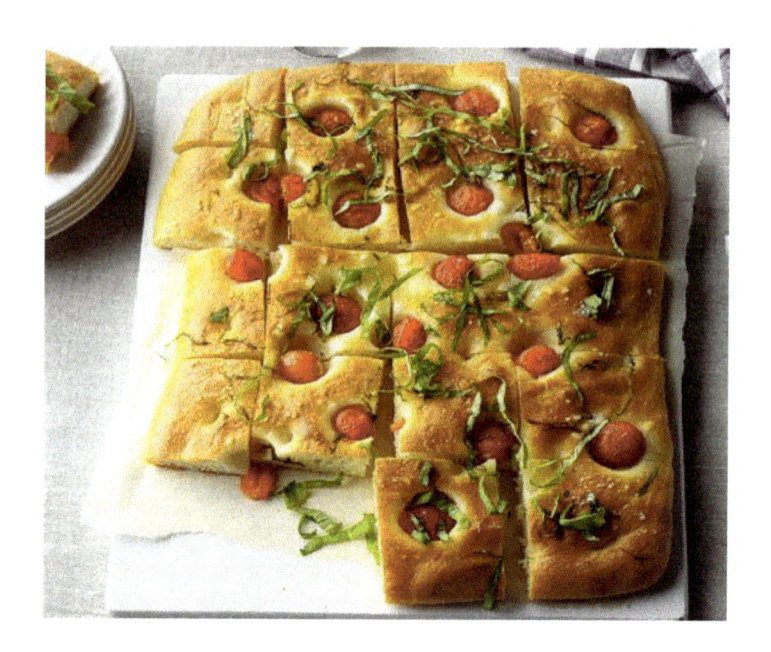

Ingredients

1 package (1/4 ounce) active dry yeast
2 cups warm 2% milk (110° to 115°)
1/4 cup canola oil
4-1/2 teaspoons sugar
1 teaspoon salt
5 to 5-1/2 cups all-purpose flour
2 cups cherry tomatoes
1/3 cup olive oil
2 tablespoons cornmeal
3 tablespoons thinly sliced fresh basil
1 teaspoon coarse salt
1/8 teaspoon pepper

Directions

In a small bowl, dissolve yeast in warm milk. In a large bowl, combine canola oil, sugar, salt, yeast mixture and 2 cups flour; beat on medium speed until smooth. Stir in enough remaining flour to form a stiff dough (dough will be sticky).

Turn dough onto a floured surface; knead until smooth and elastic, 6-8 minutes. Place in a greased bowl, turning once to grease the top. Cover and let rise in a warm place until doubled, about 45 minutes. Meanwhile, fill a large saucepan two-thirds with water; bring to a boil. Cut a shallow "X" on the bottom of each tomato. Using a slotted spoon, place tomatoes, a cup at a time, in boiling water for 30 seconds or just until skin at the "X" begins to loosen. Remove tomatoes and immediately drop into ice water. Pull off and discard skins. Place tomatoes in a small bowl; drizzle with oil.

Preheat oven to 425°. Sprinkle 2 greased baking sheets with cornmeal; set aside. Punch down dough. Turn onto a lightly floured surface. Cover; let rest 10 minutes. Divide dough in half. Shape each into a 12x8-in. rectangle and place on prepared baking sheets.

Using fingertips, press several dimples into dough. Pour tomato mixture over dough; sprinkle with basil, coarse salt and pepper. Let rise in a warm place until doubled, about 30 minutes.

Bake until golden brown, 15-18 minutes.

35. Tortellini with Tomato Spinach Cream Sauce

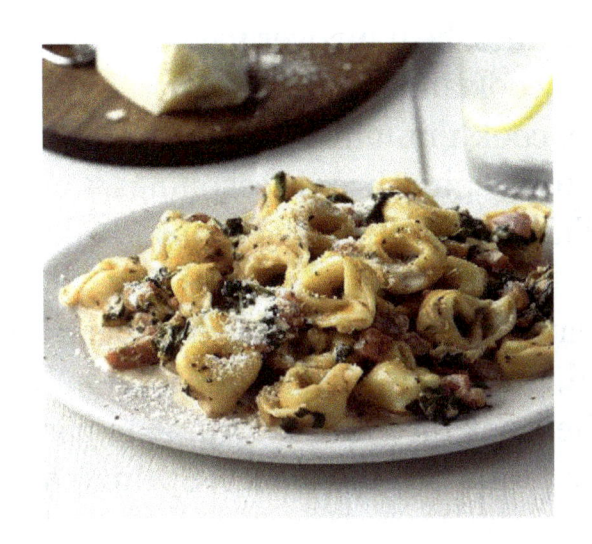

Ingredients

1 tablespoon olive oil
1 small onion, chopped
3 garlic cloves, minced
1 can (14-1/2 ounces) petite diced tomatoes, undrained
5 ounces frozen chopped spinach, thawed and squeezed dry (about 1/2 cup)
1 teaspoon dried basil
3/4 teaspoon salt
1/2 teaspoon pepper
1 cup heavy whipping cream
1 package (19 ounces) frozen cheese tortellini
1/2 cup grated Parmesan cheese

Directions

In a large skillet, heat oil over medium-high heat. Add onion; cook and stir until tender, 2-3 minutes. Add garlic; cook 1 minute longer.
Add tomatoes, spinach and seasonings. Cook and stir over medium heat until liquid is absorbed, about 3 minutes.
Stir in cream; bring to a boil. Reduce heat; simmer, uncovered, until thickened, about 10 minutes. Meanwhile, cook tortellini according to package directions; drain. Stir into sauce. Sprinkle with cheese.

36. Eggplant Parmesan

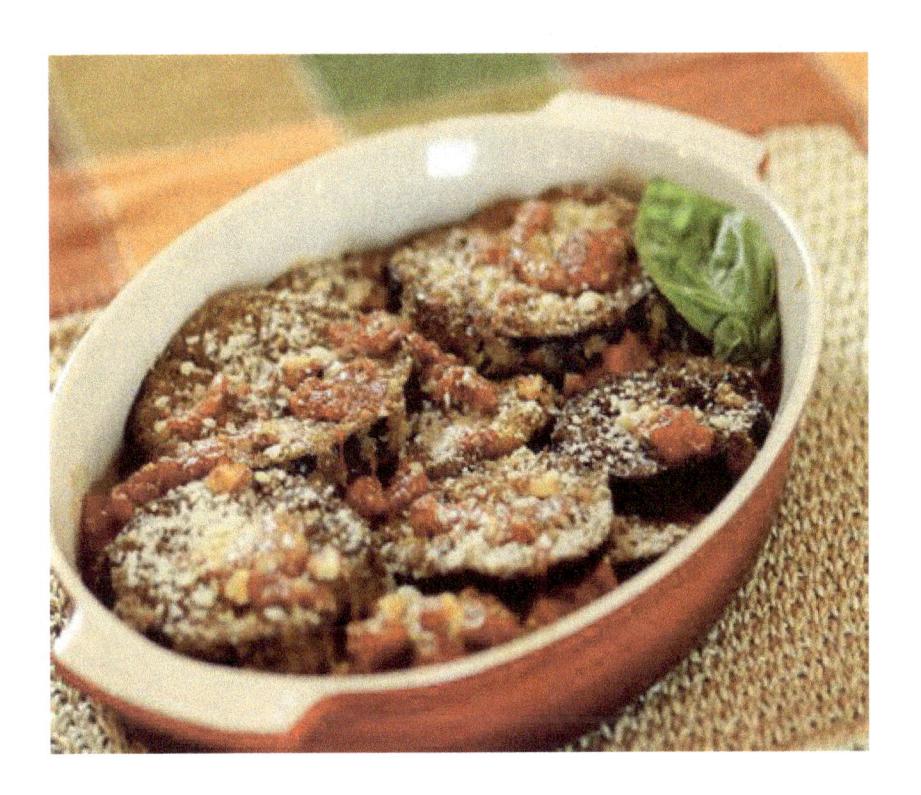

Ingredients

2 tablespoons olive oil
1 garlic clove, minced
1 small eggplant, peeled and cut into 1/4-inch slices
1 tablespoon minced fresh basil or 1 teaspoon dried basil
1 tablespoon grated Parmesan cheese
1 medium tomato, thinly sliced
1/2 cup shredded mozzarella cheese

Directions

Combine oil and garlic; brush over both sides of eggplant slices. Place on a greased baking sheet. Bake at 425° for 15 minutes; turn. Bake until golden brown, about 5 minutes longer. Cool on a wire rack. Place half of the eggplant in a greased 1-qt. baking dish. Sprinkle with half of the basil and Parmesan cheese. Arrange tomato slices over top; sprinkle with remaining basil and Parmesan. Layer with half of the mozzarella cheese and the remaining eggplant; top with remaining mozzarella. Cover and bake at 350° for 20 minutes. Uncover; bake until cheese is melted, 5-7 minutes longer. Garnish with additional basil, if desired.

37. Grilled Bruschetta

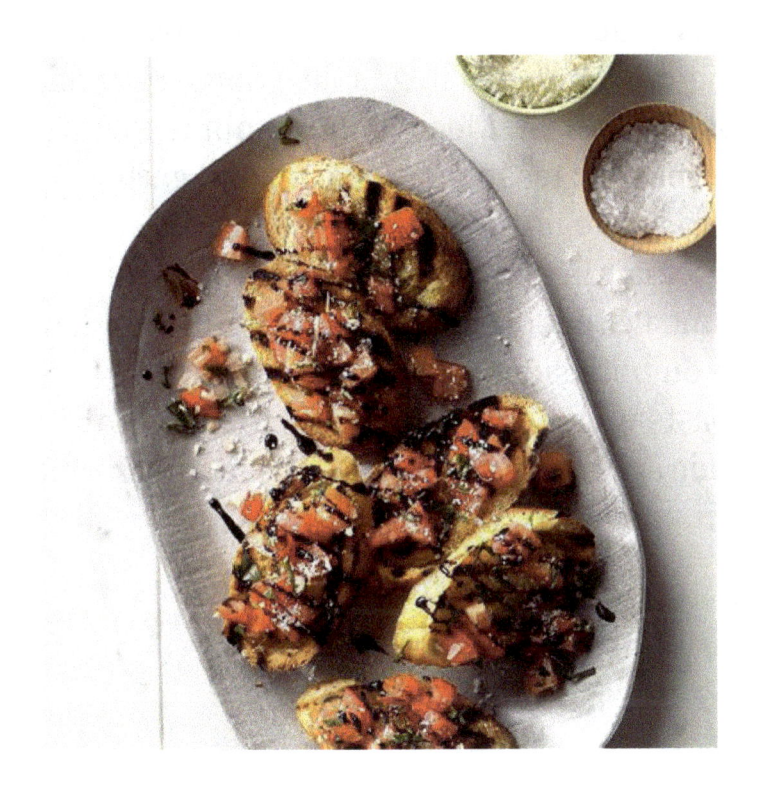

Ingredients

1/2 cup balsamic vinegar
1-1/2 cups chopped and seeded plum tomatoes
2 tablespoons finely chopped shallot
1 tablespoon minced fresh basil
2 teaspoons plus 3 tablespoons olive oil, divided
1 garlic clove, minced
16 slices French bread baguette (1/2 inch thick)
Sea salt and grated Parmesan cheese

Directions

In a small saucepan, bring vinegar to a boil; cook until liquid is reduced to 3 tablespoons, 8-10 minutes. Remove from heat. Meanwhile, combine tomatoes, shallot, basil, 2 teaspoons olive oil and garlic. Cover and refrigerate until serving.

Brush remaining oil over both sides of baguette slices. Grill, uncovered, over medium heat until golden brown on both sides.

Top toasts with tomato mixture. Drizzle with balsamic syrup; sprinkle with sea salt and Parmesan. Serve immediately.

38. Make-Ahead Spinach Manicotti

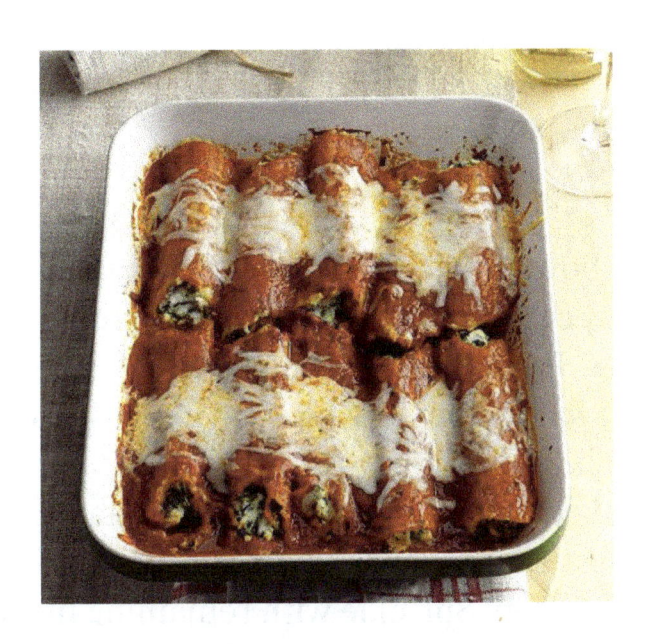

Ingredients

1 carton (15 ounces) whole-milk ricotta cheese
1 package (10 ounces) frozen chopped spinach, thawed and squeezed dry
1-1/2 cups shredded part-skim mozzarella cheese, divided
3/4 cup shredded Parmesan cheese, divided
1 large egg, lightly beaten
2 teaspoons minced fresh parsley
1/2 teaspoon onion powder
1/2 teaspoon pepper
1/8 teaspoon garlic powder
3 jars (24 ounces each) spaghetti sauce

1 cup water
1 package (8 ounces) manicotti shells

Directions

In a large bowl, mix ricotta, spinach, 1 cup mozzarella cheese, 1/4 cup Parmesan cheese, egg, parsley and seasonings. In another large bowl, mix spaghetti sauce and water; spread 1 cup into a greased 13x9-in. baking dish.
Fill uncooked manicotti shells with ricotta mixture; arrange over sauce. Pour remaining spaghetti sauce mixture over top. Sprinkle with remaining mozzarella cheese and Parmesan cheese. Refrigerate, covered, overnight.
Remove from refrigerator 30 minutes before baking. Preheat oven to 350°. Bake, uncovered, 40-50 minutes or until manicotti is tender.
Freeze option: Cover and freeze unbaked casserole. To use, partially thaw in refrigerator overnight. Remove from refrigerator 30 minutes before baking. Preheat oven to 350°. Bake casserole as directed, increasing time as necessary to heat through and for a thermometer inserted in center to read 165°.

39. Artichoke Caprese Platter

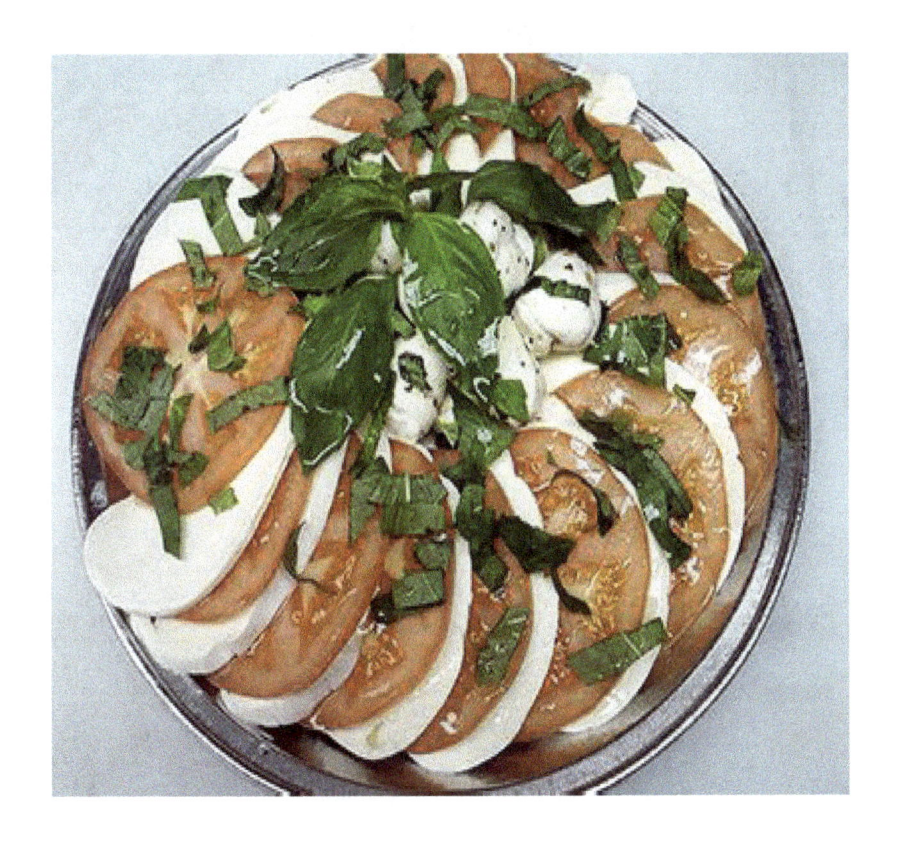

Ingredients

2 jars (7-1/2 ounces each) marinated artichoke hearts
2 tablespoons red wine vinegar
2 tablespoons olive oil
6 plum tomatoes, sliced
1 pound fresh mozzarella cheese, sliced
2 cups loosely packed fresh basil leaves
Coarsely ground pepper, optional

Directions

Drain the artichokes, reserving 1/2 cup marinade. In a small bowl, whisk vinegar, oil and the reserved marinade.

On a large serving platter, arrange the artichokes, tomatoes, mozzarella cheese and basil. Drizzle with vinaigrette. If desired, sprinkle with coarsely ground pepper.

40. Gnocchi Alfredo

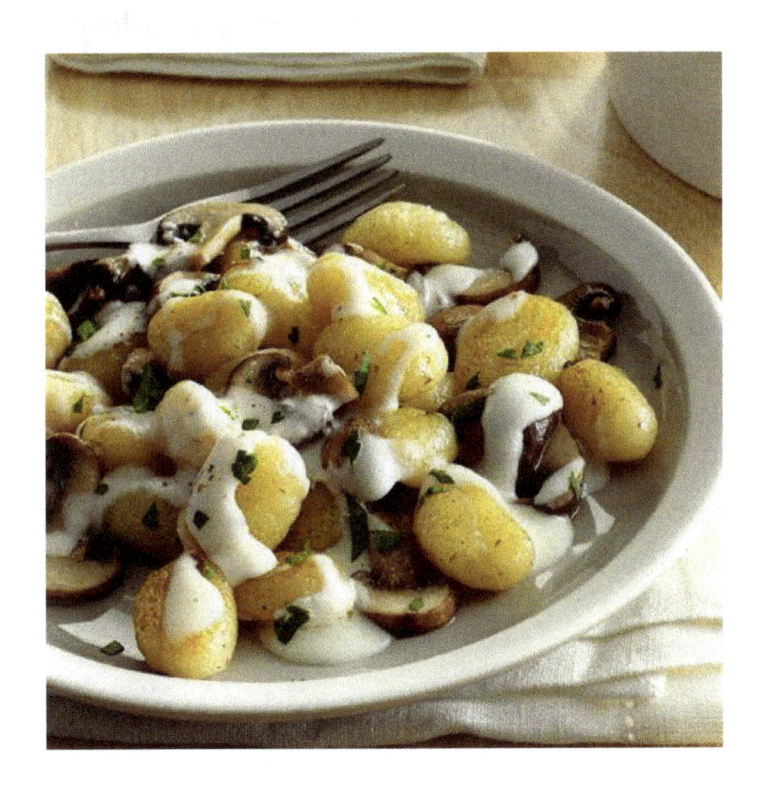

Ingredients

2 pounds potato gnocchi
3 tablespoons butter, divided
1 tablespoon plus 1-1/2 teaspoons all-purpose flour
1-1/2 cups whole milk
1/2 cup grated Parmesan cheese
Dash ground nutmeg
1/2 pound sliced baby portobello mushrooms
Minced fresh parsley, optional

Directions

Cook gnocchi according to package directions; drain. Meanwhile, in a small saucepan, melt 1 tablespoon butter. Stir in flour until smooth; gradually whisk in milk. Bring to a boil, stirring constantly; cook and stir 1-2 minutes or until thickened. Remove from heat; stir in cheese and nutmeg until blended. Keep warm. In a large heavy skillet, melt remaining butter over medium heat. Heat 5-7 minutes or until golden brown, stirring constantly. Immediately add mushrooms and gnocchi; cook and stir 4-5 minutes or until mushrooms are tender and gnocchi are lightly browned. Serve with sauce. If desired, sprinkle with parsley.

41. Creamy Italian Potato Salad

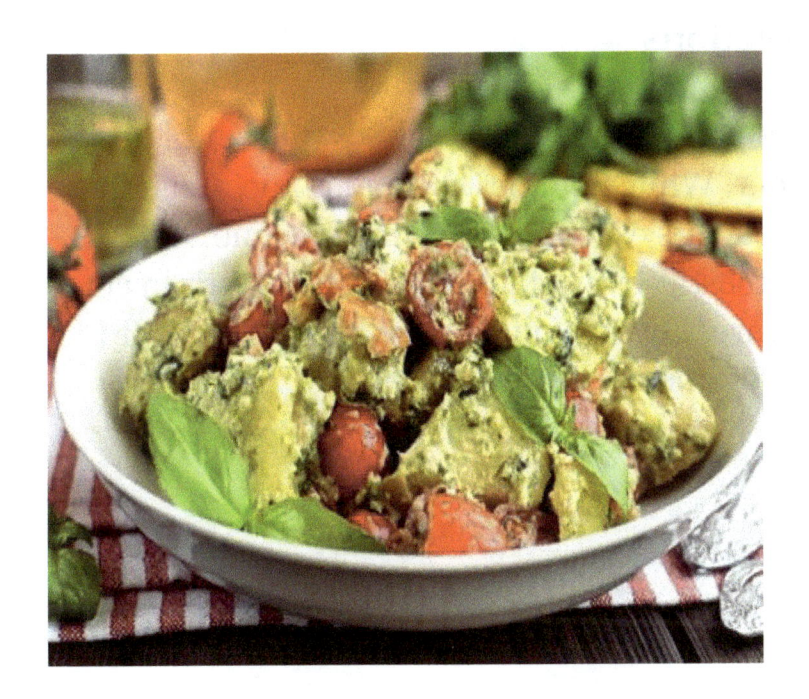

Ingredients

3 pounds red potatoes, cubed
2/3 cup grated Parmesan cheese
1 cup (9 ounces) ricotta cheese
4 garlic cloves, minced
1/2 medium red onion, sliced in thin rings
1/2 cup olive oil
6 tablespoons cider vinegar
Salt to taste
Coarsely ground pepper
1/2 cup minced fresh parsley
1/2 teaspoon dried oregano

Directions

Cook potatoes in boiling salted water until just tender. While potatoes cool, combine remaining ingredients except parsley and oregano. Drain potatoes. While potatoes are still hot, stir in cheese mixture. Cover; chill. Just before serving, stir in parsley and oregano.

42. Panzanella Pasta

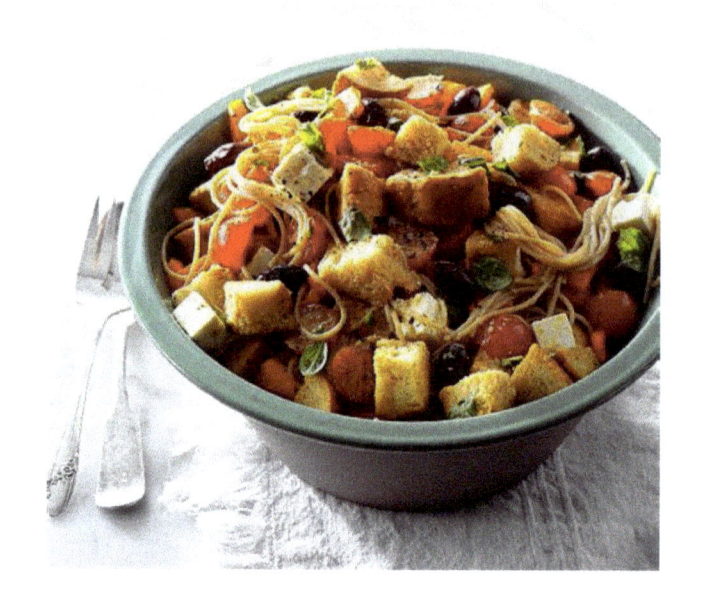

Ingredients

4 ounces uncooked whole wheat spaghetti
2 tablespoons plus 1/2 cup olive oil, divided
6 cups cubed French bread (1-inch pieces)
1/3 cup red wine vinegar
2 tablespoons Dijon mustard
1 teaspoon salt
1/2 teaspoon coarsely ground pepper
4 cups cherry tomatoes, halved
2 medium sweet yellow or orange peppers, chopped
1/2 cup pitted Greek olives
1/2 cup loosely packed basil leaves, torn

8 ounces feta or part-skim mozzarella cheese, cut into 1/2-inch cubes

Directions

Cook spaghetti according to package directions. In a large skillet, heat 2 tablespoons oil over medium-high heat. Add bread cubes; cook and stir 3-4 minutes or until toasted. Remove from heat.
In a large bowl, whisk vinegar, mustard, salt, pepper and remaining oil until blended. Add tomatoes, peppers, olives and basil; toss lightly.
Drain spaghetti and add to tomato mixture. Add toasted bread cubes and cheese; toss to combine. Serve immediately.

43. Bow Ties with Walnut-Herb Pesto

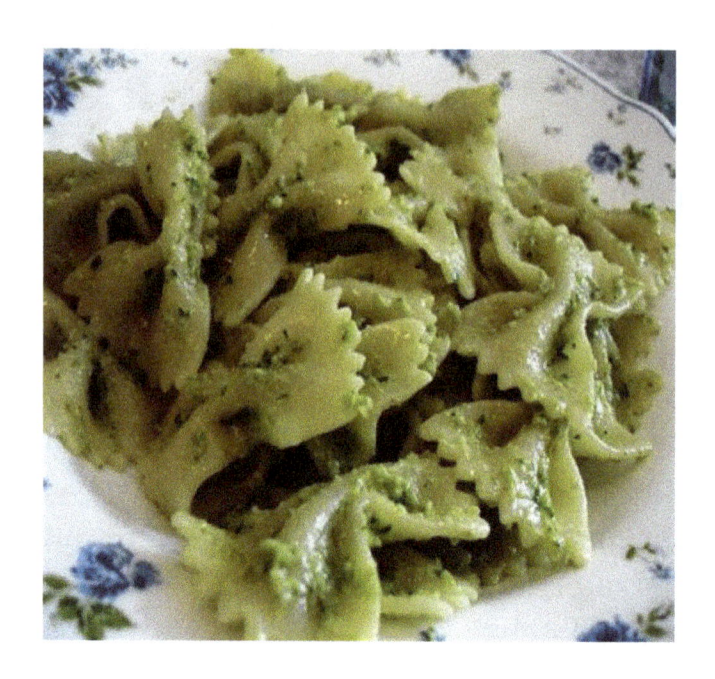

Ingredients

4 cups uncooked whole wheat bow tie pasta
1 cup fresh arugula
1/2 cup packed fresh parsley sprigs
1/2 cup loosely packed basil leaves
1/4 cup grated Parmesan cheese
1/2 teaspoon salt
1/8 teaspoon crushed red pepper flakes
1/4 cup chopped walnuts
1/3 cup olive oil
1 plum tomato, seeded and chopped

Directions

Cook pasta according to package directions. Meanwhile, place the arugula, parsley, basil, cheese, salt and pepper flakes in a food processor; cover and pulse until chopped. Add walnuts; cover and process until blended. While processing, gradually add oil in a steady stream.
Drain pasta, reserving 3 tablespoons cooking water. In a large bowl, toss pasta with pesto, tomato and reserved water.

44. Mushroom Bolognese with Whole Wheat Pasta

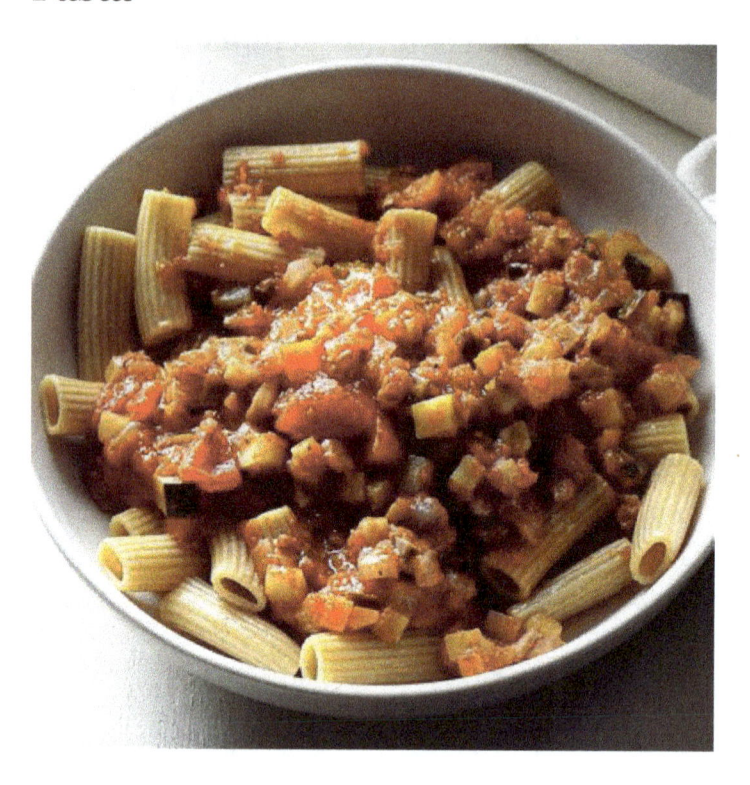

Ingredients

1 tablespoon olive oil
1 large sweet onion, finely chopped
2 medium carrots, finely chopped
1 large zucchini, finely chopped
1/2 pound baby portobello mushrooms, finely chopped
3 garlic cloves, minced
1/2 cup dry red wine or reduced-sodium chicken broth

1 can (28 ounces) crushed tomatoes, undrained
1 can (14-1/2 ounces) diced tomatoes, undrained
1/2 cup grated Parmesan cheese
1/2 teaspoon dried oregano
1/2 teaspoon pepper
1/8 teaspoon crushed red pepper flakes
Dash ground nutmeg
4-1/2 cups uncooked whole wheat rigatoni

Directions

In a 6-qt. stockpot coated with cooking spray, heat oil over medium-high heat. Add onion and carrots; cook and stir until tender. Add zucchini, mushrooms and garlic; cook and stir until tender. Stir in wine; bring to a boil; cook until liquid is almost evaporated. Stir in crushed and diced tomatoes, cheese and seasonings; bring to a boil. Reduce heat; simmer, covered, 25-30 minutes or until slightly thickened. Cook rigatoni according to package directions; drain. Serve with sauce.

45. Italian-Style Pizzas

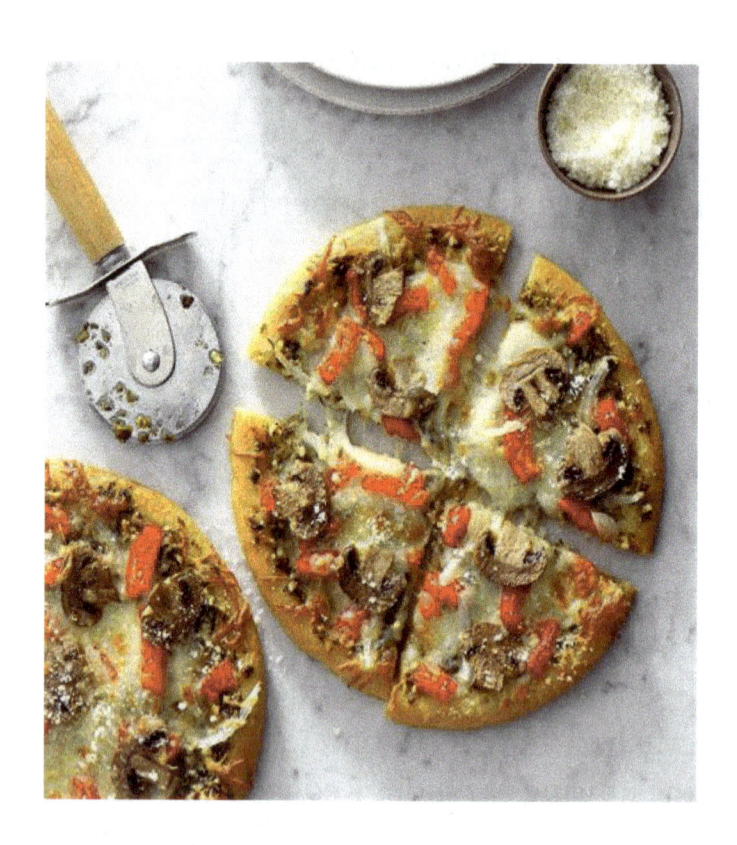

Ingredients

2 prebaked mini pizza crusts
1/2 cup prepared pesto
2/3 cup shredded part-skim mozzarella cheese
1/2 cup sliced sweet onion
1/2 cup thinly sliced fresh mushrooms
1/4 cup roasted sweet red peppers, drained
2 tablespoons grated Parmesan cheese

Directions

Place crusts on an ungreased baking sheet; spread with pesto. Layer with mozzarella cheese, onion, mushrooms and peppers; sprinkle with Parmesan cheese. Bake at 400° until cheese is melted, 10-12 minutes.

46. Creamy Pasta Primavera

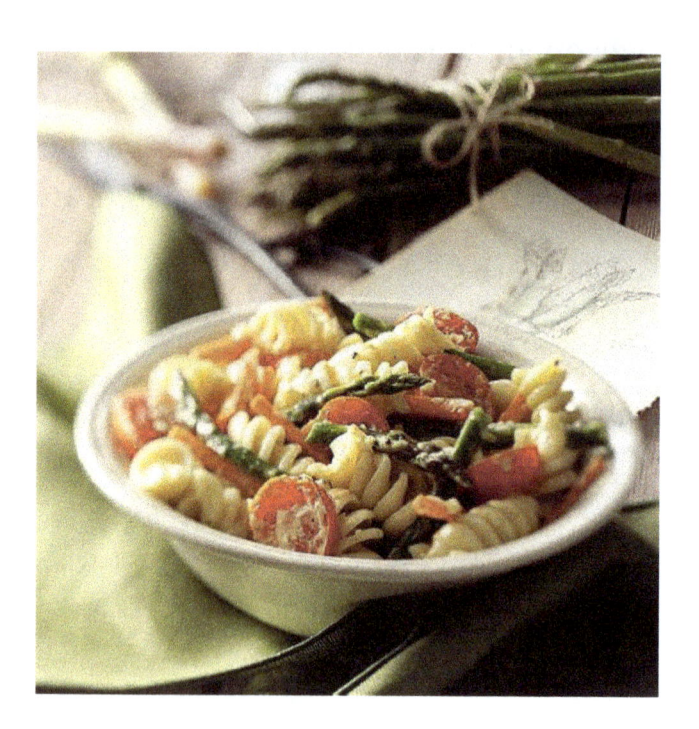

Ingredients

2 cups uncooked gemelli or spiral pasta
1 pound fresh asparagus, trimmed and cut into 2-inch pieces
3 medium carrots, shredded
2 teaspoons canola oil
2 cups cherry tomatoes, halved
1 garlic clove, minced
1/2 cup grated Parmesan cheese
1/2 cup heavy whipping cream
1/4 teaspoon pepper

Directions

Cook pasta according to package directions. In a large skillet over medium-high heat, saute asparagus and carrots in oil until crisp-tender. Add tomatoes and garlic; cook 1 minute longer.
Stir in the cheese, cream and pepper. Drain pasta; toss with asparagus mixture.

47. Tuscan Portobello Stew

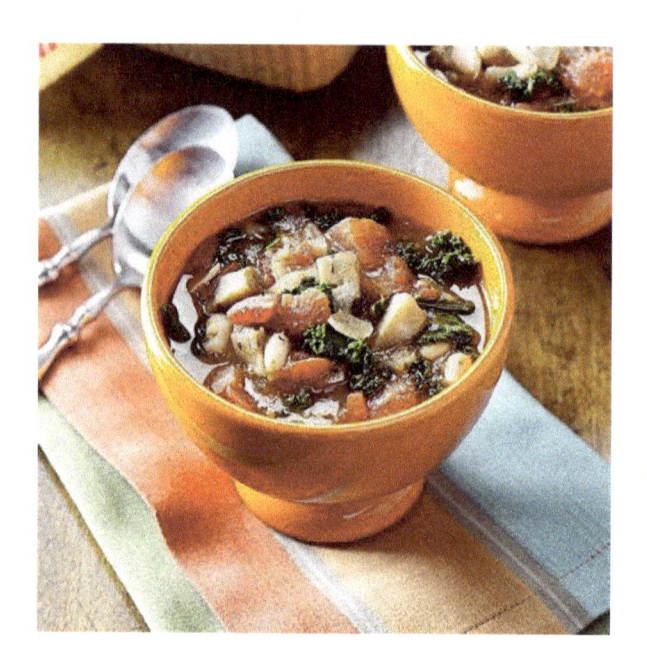

Ingredients

2 large portobello mushrooms, coarsely chopped
1 medium onion, chopped
3 garlic cloves, minced
2 tablespoons olive oil
1/2 cup white wine or vegetable broth
1 can (28 ounces) diced tomatoes, undrained
2 cups chopped fresh kale
1 bay leaf
1 teaspoon dried thyme
1/2 teaspoon dried basil
1/2 teaspoon dried rosemary, crushed

1/4 teaspoon salt
1/4 teaspoon pepper
2 cans (15 ounces each) cannellini beans, rinsed and drained

Directions

In a large skillet, saute the mushrooms, onion and garlic in oil until tender. Add the wine. Bring to a boil; cook until liquid is reduced by half. Stir in the tomatoes, kale and seasonings. Bring to a boil. Reduce heat; cover and simmer for 8-10 minutes. Add beans; heat through. Discard bay leaf.

48. Slow-Cooker Caponata

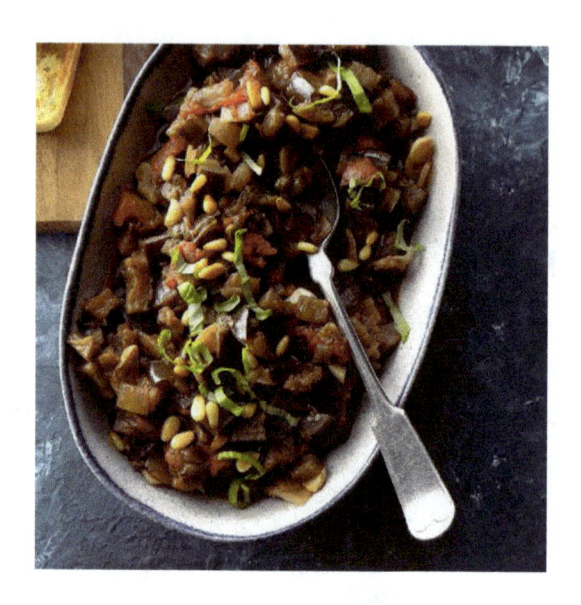

Ingredients

2 medium eggplants, cut into 1/2-inch pieces
1 medium onion, chopped
1 can (14-1/2 ounces) diced tomatoes, undrained
12 garlic cloves, sliced
1/2 cup dry red wine
3 tablespoons olive oil
2 tablespoons red wine vinegar
4 teaspoons capers, undrained
5 bay leaves
1-1/2 teaspoons salt
1/4 teaspoon coarsely ground pepper

French bread baguette slices, toasted
Optional: Fresh basil leaves, toasted pine nuts and additional olive oil

Directions

Place first 11 ingredients in a 6-qt. slow cooker (do not stir). Cook, covered, on high for 3 hours. Stir gently; replace cover. Cook on high 2 hours longer or until vegetables are tender. Cool slightly; discard bay leaves. Serve with toasted baguette slices, adding toppings as desired.

49. Gnocchi with Mushrooms and Onion

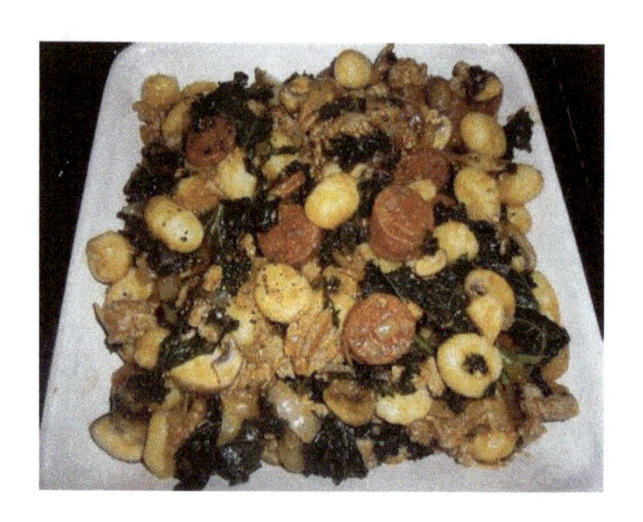

Ingredients

1 package (16 ounces) potato gnocchi
1/2 pound sliced fresh mushrooms
3/4 cup chopped sweet onion
1/4 cup butter, cubed
1/4 teaspoon salt
1/4 teaspoon Italian seasoning
1/4 teaspoon crushed red pepper flakes
Grated Parmesan cheese

Directions

Cook gnocchi according to package directions. Meanwhile, in a large cast-iron skillet, saute mushrooms and onion in butter until tender.

Drain gnocchi. Add the gnocchi, salt, Italian seasoning and pepper flakes to the skillet; heat through. Sprinkle with cheese.

50. Quinoa Arancini

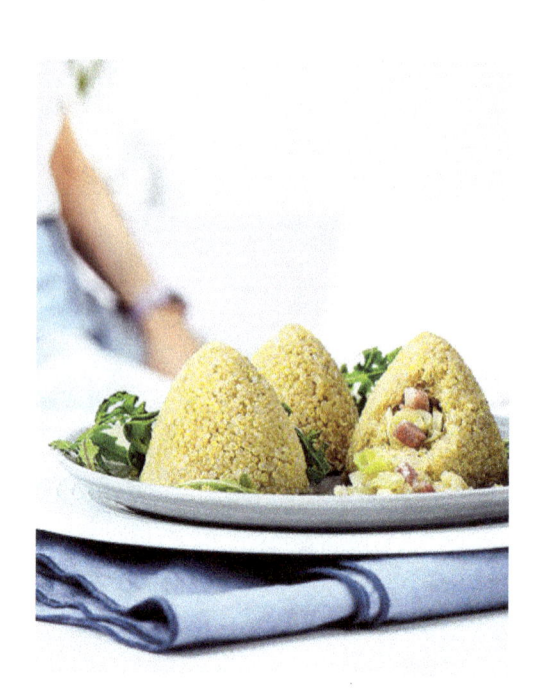

Ingredients

1 package (9 ounces) ready-to-serve quinoa or 1-3/4 cups cooked quinoa
2 large eggs, lightly beaten, divided use
1 cup seasoned bread crumbs, divided
1/4 cup shredded Parmesan cheese
1 tablespoon olive oil
2 tablespoons minced fresh basil or 2 teaspoons dried basil
1/2 teaspoon garlic powder

1/2 teaspoon salt
1/8 teaspoon pepper
6 cubes part-skim mozzarella cheese (3/4 inch each)
Cooking spray
Warmed pasta sauce, optional

Directions

Preheat oven to 425°. Prepare quinoa according to package directions. Stir in 1 egg, 1/2 cup bread crumbs, Parmesan cheese, oil, basil and seasonings. Divide into 6 portions. Shape each portion around a cheese cube to cover completely, forming a ball. Place remaining egg and 1/2 cup bread crumbs in separate shallow bowls. Dip quinoa balls in egg, then roll in bread crumbs. Place on a greased in baking pan; spritz with cooking spray. Bake until golden brown, 15-20 minutes. If desired, serve with pasta sauce.

Conclusion

My goal was to make these recipes easy to prepare, but above all tasty to the palate, so we hope you enjoyed them.

In this book, you were able to learn about several Italian recipes that you might not have otherwise learned about in other books.

I have created these recipes for those who are already experts but also for those who are beginners and are approaching this type of cooking for the first time, so train often and get familiar with the recipes, you will see that in addition to having advantages at the physical level you will increase your culinary skills.

Thanks for choosing me, see you at the next book.

CPSIA information can be obtained
at www.ICGtesting.com
Printed in the USA
LVHW010140160621
690356LV00011B/1032